Do Children Have Rights?

Do Children Have Rights?

Other books in the At Issue series:

At ✳ Issue

Do Children Have Rights?

Jamuna Carroll, *Book Editor*

Bruce Glassman, *Vice President*
Bonnie Szumski, *Publisher*
Helen Cothran, *Managing Editor*

GREENHAVEN PRESS
An imprint of Thomson Gale, a part of The Thomson Corporation

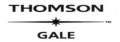
THOMSON
GALE

Detroit • New York • San Francisco • San Diego • New Haven, Conn.
Waterville, Maine • London • Munich

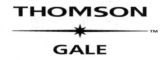

For more information, contact
Greenhaven Press
27500 Drake Rd.
Farmington Hills, MI 48331-3535
Or you can visit our Internet site at http://www.gale.com

Greenhaven Press anthologies primarily consist of previously published material taken from a variety of sources, including periodicals, books, scholarly journals, newspapers, government documents, and position papers from private and public organizations. These original sources are often edited for length and to ensure their accessibility for a young adult audience. The anthology editors also change the original titles of these works in order to clearly present the main thesis of each viewpoint and to explicitly indicate the opinion presented in the viewpoint. These alterations are made in consideration of both the reading and comprehension levels of a young adult audience. Every effort is made to ensure that Greenhaven Press accurately reflects the original intent of the authors included in this anthology.

LIBRARY OF CONGRESS CATALOGING-IN-PUBLICATION DATA

Do children have rights? / Jamuna Carroll, book editor.
    p. cm. — (At issue)
  Includes bibliographical references and index.
  ISBN 0-7377-2366-1 (lib. : alk. paper) — ISBN 0-7377-2367-X (pbk. : alk. paper)
    1. Children's rights. 2. Children—Legal status, laws, etc. I. Carroll, Jamuna.
  II. At issue (San Diego, Calif.)
  HQ789.D62 2006
  323.3'52—dc22   2005046327

Printed in the United States of America

Contents

Introduction

Circulating in some African and Asian countries is the dangerously false belief that an AIDS patient can be cured by having sex with a virgin. Tragically, some men with AIDS, mainly in South Africa, have persuaded adolescent girls to have sex with them and have raped infants and children as well. Although these men believe that having unprotected intercourse with a virgin is healing, it only exposes the girl to an incurable disease with which 30 million Africans are currently afflicted. As this example clearly demonstrates, misinformation and naïveté about AIDS directly fuels its spread. The United Nations Children's Fund (UNICEF), which has identified education as an invaluable tool for curbing the epidemic, asserts, "All people have a right to know what HIV [the virus that causes AIDS] is, how it is transmitted and how to prevent infection." Likewise, Human Rights Watch maintains that access to information about AIDS "is not simply a public health imperative—it is a human right." Numerous world organizations, in fact, have charged that the violation of children's right to receive accurate information about the disease is contributing to its rapid proliferation in Africa.

Over 6 million Africans under twenty-five years of age live with AIDS or HIV. This alarming statistic underscores the importance of early prevention education. According to the 1997 World AIDS Campaign:

> The [AIDS] epidemic . . . casts its biggest shadow on the hundreds of millions of uninfected children who face a lifetime risk of HIV infection as they grow into adulthood. . . . Governments' responsibility . . . extends to fulfilling the rights of children such as to information, education and services.

As imperative as education is in the global battle against AIDS, fewer than half of young women surveyed in twenty-six countries (mainly in Africa) could identify all three ways in which the disease can be averted. Human rights groups attribute this lack of knowledge to certain school-based AIDS education programs that teach children only two of the three prevention methods: abstinence until marriage and being committed to one sexual partner, with an emphasis on abstinence. The use of condoms to prevent AIDS is not discussed in many countries' school curricula. This is because condoms are not 100 percent effective, government leaders explain, and because promoting condom use may encourage youths to have sex. However, the United Nations Committee on the Rights of the Child retorts, "Effective HIV/AIDS prevention requires States to refrain from censoring, withholding or intentionally misrepresenting health-related information, including sexual education and information." Children, world organizations contend, have a right to know that condoms can keep them from acquiring a fatal illness.

Another controversial aspect of these sex education programs is their suggestion that youths need not worry about AIDS once they are married. Marriage, caution welfare organizations, does not necessarily shield people from the disease. In Uganda, for example, girls who marry before the age of eighteen generally marry men who have been sexually active for years, often without using condoms. Consequently, even those who abstain until marriage may be exposed to HIV by their new spouse. Polygamy and adultery also contribute to new infections in Africa. In both situations, men may contract HIV from—and spread it to—prostitutes, their girlfriends, and their multiple wives. A Ugandan woman sums up this increasingly common problem: "I got HIV in marriage. I was faithful in my relationship." Adrienne Germain of the International Women's Health Coalition adds, "Most African women who have AIDS are monogamous and married." Several groups accuse AIDS educators in Africa of ignoring these facts by continuing to champion abstinence until marriage as the best prevention.

Alleged deficiencies in AIDS education programs especially affect children whose parents have died of the disease, many experts contend. In sub-Saharan Africa alone there are 11 million AIDS orphans. With no relatives to support and protect them, many become prostitutes. Unaware that using condoms could ward off the disease, young sex workers are likely to become infected with HIV. Human Rights Watch reports:

> As AIDS impoverishes families, young people—especially young girls—are likely to be withdrawn from school and forced into exploitative situations to survive. Ignorance and denial fuel HIV even further, leaving young people without the critical in-

formation that could help them prevent infection.
. . . The phenomenon of girls having sex with older men, often out of economic need, is thought to account for a significant number of new HIV infections in Uganda.

In response to the pandemic, the international community has held conferences on how best to combat AIDS. During a special session on HIV/AIDS in 2001, for instance, the United Nations vowed to

ensure that . . . by 2010 at least 95 percent of young men and women aged 15 to 24 have access to the information, education—including peer education and youth-specific HIV education—and services necessary to develop the life skills required to reduce their vulnerability to HIV infection.

A point on which many groups concur is that adolescents must be guaranteed their right to access all available AIDS information before the aspiration of an AIDS-free world can be realized. However, they are opposed by some governments and organizations that believe instructing youths about condom use would increase teen sexual activity and actually spread AIDS. Agreement regarding the other rights of children is often as difficult to reach. This anthology, *At Issue: Do Children Have Rights?*, provides a forum where authors voice clashing opinions on the human and constitutional rights of minors in areas such as child labor, voting, and abortion.

1

Children Have the Same Rights as Adults

United Nations Children's Fund

United Nations Children's Fund (UNICEF) is a world organization that works with decision makers, families, and other organizations to advance children's rights everywhere.

Children have the same civil, political, economic, social, and cultural rights as do adults, for human rights apply to all people no matter what their age. Every country in the world but two (the United States and Somalia) has signaled its support of children's rights by ratifying the Convention on the Rights of the Child, an international human rights treaty. The convention declares that all youths worldwide have the right to survival, full participation in their family and society, and protection from exploitation and abuse. Specifically, all minors—regardless of sex, religion, or social origin—deserve the right to health care, education, social services, and free expression. Widespread acceptance of the declaration indicates global agreement that children are their own beings and are not merely the property of their parents.

> "A century that began with children having virtually no rights is ending with children having the most powerful legal instrument that not only recognizes but protects their human rights."
> —Carol Bellamy, UNICEF Executive Director

United Nations Children's Fund, "Convention on the Rights of the Child," www.unhchr.ch/html/menu3/b/k2crc.htm. Copyright © by United Nations Publications. Reproduced by permission.

The human rights of children, and the standards to which all governments must aspire in realizing these rights for all children, are most concisely and fully articulated in one international human rights treaty: the Convention on the Rights of the Child. The Convention is the most universally accepted human rights instrument in history—it has been ratified by every country in the world except two—and therefore uniquely places children centre-stage in the quest for the universal application of human rights. By ratifying this instrument, national governments have committed themselves to protecting and ensuring children's rights and they have agreed to hold themselves accountable for this commitment before the international community.

The Preservation of Children's Rights

Built on varied legal systems and cultural traditions, the Convention on the Rights of the Child is a universally agreed set of non-negotiable standards and obligations. It spells out the basic human rights that children everywhere—without discrimination—have: the right to survival; to develop to the fullest; to protection from harmful influences, abuse and exploitation; and to participate fully in family, cultural and social life. Every right spelled out in the Convention is inherent to the human dignity and harmonious development of every child. The Convention protects children's rights by setting standards in health care, education and legal, civil and social services. These standards are benchmarks against which progress can be assessed. States that are party to the Convention are obliged to develop and undertake all actions and policies in the light of the best interests of the child.

> *Children everywhere . . . have: the right to survival; to develop to the fullest; to protection from harmful influences, abuse and exploitation; and to participate fully in family, cultural and social life.*

The Convention on the Rights of the Child is the first legally binding international instrument to incorporate the full range of human rights—civil and political rights as well as economic, social and cultural rights. Two Optional Protocols, on the involvement of children in armed conflict and on the sale of children, child prostitution and child pornography, were adopted to strengthen the provisions of the Convention in these areas. They entered into force, respectively on 12 February and 18 January 2002.

All Children Have Rights

"Human rights are inscribed in the hearts of people; they were there long before lawmakers drafted their first proclamation."
—Mary Robinson, former United Nations High Commissioner for Human Rights

Prior to the Convention on the Rights of the Child, human rights standards applicable to all members of the human family had been expressed in legal instruments such as covenants, conventions and declarations, as did standards relating to the specific concerns of children. But it was only in 1989 that the standards concerning children were brought together in a single legal instrument, approved by the international community and spelling out in an unequivocal manner the rights to which every child is entitled, regardless of where born or to whom, regardless of sex, religion, or social origin. The body of rights enumerated in the Convention are the rights of all children *everywhere.*

> *Children living in rural areas may have fewer opportunities to obtain an education . . . [or to access] health services than children living in cities. . . . Such disparities [are] a violation of human rights.*

The idea of *everywhere* is important. In too many countries, children's lives are plagued by armed conflict, child labour, sexual exploitation and other human rights violations. Elsewhere, for example, children living in rural areas may have fewer opportunities to obtain an education of good quality or may have less access to health services than children living in cities. The

Convention states that such disparities—within societies—are also a violation of human rights. In calling on governments to ensure the human rights of all children, the Convention seeks to correct these kinds of inequities.

Some people assume that the rights of children born in wealthy nations—where schools, hospitals and juvenile justice systems are in place—are never violated, that these children have no need for the protection and care called for in the Convention. But that is far from the truth. To varying degrees, at least *some* children in *all* nations face unemployment, homelessness, violence, poverty and other issues that dramatically affect their lives.

Human Rights Belong to Each of Us Equally

All of us are born with human rights—a principle the Convention on the Rights of the Child makes very clear. Human rights are not something a richer person gives to a poorer person; nor are they owned by a select few and given to others as a mere favour or gift. They belong to each and every one of us equally. Children living in developing countries have the same rights as children in wealthy countries. And human rights apply to all age groups—they do not magically begin with a child's passage into adulthood, nor do they stop when the mandate of the Convention ceases on the child's reaching the age of 18.

The Convention places equal emphasis on all of the rights for children. There is no such thing as a 'small' right and no hierarchy of human rights. All the rights enumerated in the Convention—the civil and political rights as well as the economic, social and cultural rights—are indivisible and interrelated, with a focus on the child as a whole.

> *" Human rights apply to all age groups—they do not magically begin with a child's passage into adulthood. "*

This indivisibility of rights is key to interpreting the Convention. Decisions with regard to any one right must be made in the light of all the other rights in the Convention. For example, it is not sufficient to ensure that a child receives immunization and health care, only for that child on reaching the age of 14 to be sold into bonded labour or conscripted into an army. It is not enough to guarantee the right to education, only to fail to ensure that all children are enrolled in school and can go to school equally, regardless of gender or economic class.

A New Vision

The Convention on the Rights of the Child reflects a new vision of the child. Children are neither the property of their parents nor are they helpless objects of charity. They are human beings and are the subject of their own rights. The Convention offers a vision of the child as an individual *and* as a member of a family and community, with rights and responsibilities appropriate to his or her age and stage of development. By recognizing children's rights in this way, the Convention firmly sets the focus on the whole child.

> **"***Children are neither the property of their parents nor are they helpless objects of charity. They are human beings and are the subject of their own rights.***"**

The Convention on the Rights of the Child:

Reinforces fundamental human dignity. Because of its near-universal acceptance by the community of nations, the Convention on the Rights of the Child has brought into sharp focus for the first time the fundamental human dignity of all children and the urgency of ensuring their well-being and development. Considered the most powerful legal instrument for the recognition and protection of children's human rights, the Convention draws on the following unique combination of strengths.

Highlights and defends the family's role in children's lives. In the preamble and in article 5, article 10 and article 18, the Convention on the Rights of the Child specifically refers to the family as the fundamental group of society and the natural environment for the growth and well-being of its members, particularly children. Under the Convention, States are obliged to respect parents' primary responsibility for providing care and guidance for their children and to support parents in this regard, providing material assistance and support programmes. States are also obliged to prevent children from being separated from their families unless the separation is judged necessary for the child's best interests.

Seeks respect for children—but not at the expense of the human rights or responsibilities of others. The Convention on the Rights of the Child confirms that children have a right to express their views and to have their views taken seriously and given due weight—but it does not state that children's views are the only ones to be considered. The Convention also explicitly states that children have a responsibility to respect the rights of others, especially those of parents. The Convention emphasizes the need to respect children's "evolving capacities," but does not give children the right to make decisions for themselves at too young an age. This is rooted in the common-sense concept that the child's path from total dependence to adulthood is gradual.

> *[Under the Convention,] child rights standards are no longer merely an aspiration but, rather, are nationally binding on States.*

Endorses the principle of non-discrimination. The principle of non-discrimination is included in all the basic human rights instruments and has been carefully defined by the bodies responsible for monitoring their implementation. The Convention on the Rights of the Child states frequently that States need to identify the most vulnerable and disadvantaged children within their borders and take affirmative action to ensure that the rights of these children are realized and protected.

Establishes clear obligations. Prior to or shortly after ratifying the Convention on the Rights of the Child, States are required to bring their national legislation into line with its provisions—except where the national standards are already higher. In this way, child rights standards are no longer merely an aspiration but, rather, are nationally binding on States. Ratification also makes States publicly and internationally accountable for their actions through the process in which States report on the Convention's implementation. At the centre of the monitoring process is the Committee on the Rights of the Child, an independent, elected committee whose members are of "high moral standing" and are experts in the field of human rights.

A Binding National Commitment

"The Convention is not only a visionary document. We are reminded daily that it is an agreement that works—and its utility can be seen in the everyday use to which I have seen it increasingly being put by country after country, in policy, in practice and in law."

—Carol Bellamy, UNICEF Executive
Director, Statement to the UNICEF
Executive Board, September 1998

The Convention on the Rights of the Child was carefully drafted over the course of 10 years (1979–1989) with the input of representatives from all societies, all religions and all cultures. A working group made up of members of the United Nations Commission on Human Rights, independent experts and observer delegations of non-member governments, non-governmental organizations (NGOs) and UN [United Nations] agencies was charged with the drafting. NGOs involved in the drafting represented a range of issues—from various legal perspectives to concerns about the protection of the family.

> *Capital punishment or life imprisonment without the possibility of release is explicitly prohibited for those under age 18.*

The Convention reflects this global consensus and, in a very short period of time, it has become the most widely accepted human rights treaty ever. It has been ratified by 192 countries; only two countries have not ratified: The United States and Somalia, which have signalled their intention to ratify by formally signing the Convention. . . .

The Convention on the Rights of the Child outlines in 41 articles the human rights to be respected and protected for every child under the age of 18 years and requires that these rights are implemented in the light of the Convention's guiding principles.

Articles 42–45 cover the obligation of States Parties to disseminate the Convention's principles and provisions to adults and children; the implementation of the Convention and monitoring of progress towards the realization of child rights through States Parties' obligations; and the reporting responsibilities of States Parties.

The final clauses (articles 46–54) cover the processes of accession and ratification by States Parties; the Convention's entry into force; and the depositary function of the Secretary-General of the United Nations.

In May 2000 two Optional Protocols to the Convention were adopted by the General Assembly.

Definition of the Child

The Convention on the Rights of the Child defines as children all human beings under the age of 18, unless the relevant national laws recognize an earlier age of majority. The Convention emphasizes that States substituting an earlier age for specific purposes must do so in the context of the Convention's guiding principles—of non-discrimination, best interests of the child, maximum survival and development and participation of children. In reporting to the Committee on the Rights of the Child, States Parties must indicate whether national legislation differs from the Convention with regard to the defining ages of childhood.

While in some cases States are simply obliged to be consistent in setting benchmark ages—for example, in defining the age for admission to employment or for completion of compulsory education—in other cases, the Convention sets a clear upper benchmark:

- Capital punishment or life imprisonment without the possibility of release is explicitly prohibited for those under age 18.
- While recruitment into the armed forces or direct participation in hostilities is expressly prohibited for those under age 15 according to article 38 of the Convention, an Optional Protocol to the Convention on the involvement of children in armed conflict was adopted by the General Assembly on 25 May 2000, which raises to 18 years the age of participation in hostilities and forced recruitment of

children into armed forces. The United Nations has also set minimum age requirements for United Nations peacekeepers.

States are also free to refer in national legislation to ages over 18 as the upper benchmark in defining the child. In such instances and others—where national or international law sets child rights standards that are higher than those in the Convention on the Rights of the Child—the higher standards always prevail. This ensures that situations do not arise where Convention standards undermine any national provisions that are "more conducive to the realization of the rights of the child."

2

Children Should Not Have the Same Rights as Adults

Patrick F. Fagan

A former deputy assistant secretary of Health and Human Services, Patrick F. Fagan is now a research fellow in family and cultural issues at the conservative Heritage Foundation.

Children's liberties should not come at the expense of parents' rights. By affording youths numerous human and legal rights, the United Nations' Convention on the Rights of the Child (CRC) undermines the authority of nations and parents. The treaty guarantees children privacy, freedom of expression, freedom of association, and freedom of peaceful assembly, all of which may run counter to parents' right to raise their children as they see fit and may infringe on the right of countries to uphold their unique cultural practices. Conceivably, if children are granted all of the rights listed in the CRC, they could prevent their parents from blocking Internet pornography on their computers as well as challenge their parents in court. Another preposterous suggestion of the convention is that children be allowed to seek medical attention—such as gaining access to contraceptives or abortion services—without the knowledge of their parents.

Using the political cover of international treaties that promote women's and children's rights, the social policy sector of the United Nations [U.N.]—specifically, committees that

Patrick F. Fagan, "How U.N. Conventions on Women's and Children's Rights Undermine Family, Religion, and Sovereignty," *Heritage Foundation Backgrounder*, February 5, 2001. Copyright © 2001 by The Heritage Foundation. Reproduced by permission.

oversee implementation of U.N. treaties in social policy areas and the special-interest groups assisting them—is urging countries to change their domestic laws and national constitutions to adopt policies that ultimately will affect women and children adversely.

This is a troubling agenda for an organization that proclaims, in its Universal Declaration of Human Rights, that "The family is the natural and fundamental group unit of society and is entitled to protection by society and the state." The United Nations historically has included in treaties and documents language affirming a nation's right to determine its cultural norms and practices. The U.N. Charter itself states that "Nothing contained [herein] shall authorize the United Nations to intervene in matters which are essentially within the domestic jurisdiction of any state or shall require the Members to submit such matters to settlement under the present Charter." And a 1960 General Assembly Resolution states that "All peoples have an inalienable right to complete freedom, the exercise of their sovereignty and the integrity of their national territory."

> *The freedom of parents to raise their own children, to shape their behaviors, and to safeguard their moral upbringing will be a relic of past centuries.*

But the U.N.'s long-standing respect for the right of sovereign nations to set their own domestic policies has yielded to a new countercultural agenda espoused in U.N. committee reports and documents, particularly those relating to the implementation of the Convention on the Rights of the Child (CRC). . . .

Expanding Children's Rights

If the U.N. committees have their way, the freedom of parents to raise their own children, to shape their behaviors, and to safeguard their moral upbringing will be a relic of past centuries—despite such clear articulation of parents' rights in the Universal Declaration of Human Rights as the following: "Parents have a prior right to choose the kind of education that shall be given to their children." That almost all cultures and religions have protected the time-honored role of parents in forming the character of children does not deter the U.N. from seeking changes in domestic laws to bypass parents on matters dealing with their children.

> *The [United Nations] is suggesting that the state create some entity . . . that enables children in Belize to challenge their parents' parenting in court.*

The U.N. committees are urging states to give minor children:
- The *right to privacy,* even in the household;
- The *right to professional counseling* without parental consent or guidance;
- The *full right to abortion* and contraceptives, even when that would violate the parents' ethics and desires;
- The *right to full freedom of expression* at home and in school;
- The *legal mechanisms* to challenge in court their parents' authority in the home.

For example, the U.N. Committee on the Rights of the Child recommends to the Japanese government that it "guarantee the child's right to privacy, especially in the family." Such a measure would establish legal and structural wedges between parents and their children in the home. Normally, when children rebel against their parents, society frowns. Yet the U.N. is attempting to put in place, in policy and law, structures that foster this type of rebellion.

Among the broad "rights" of children articulated in the CRC are freedom of expression; freedom to receive and impart all information and ideas, either orally, in writing, or in print, in the form of art, or through any other media of the child's choice; freedom of association; and freedom of peaceful assembly. The language of the treaty could be interpreted to prohibit parents, for example, from putting software on their children's computers to filter out pornography if their children opposed their intervention. Once this "right" is embedded in domestic law, children could easily gain access to legal help from NGOs [nongovernmental organizations] or government agencies to challenge their parents in court.

Counseling Youths Without
Their Parents' Knowledge

Indeed, the U.N. committee report to Belize recommends that the government set up legal mechanisms to help children challenge their parents, including making an "independent child-friendly mechanism" accessible to children "to deal with complaints of violations of their rights and to provide remedies for such violations." In other words, the CRC committee is suggesting that the state create some entity to supervise parents, a structure that enables children in Belize to challenge their parents' parenting in court. Then the CRC committee goes even further: Its report asserts that it is "concerned that the law does not allow children, particularly adolescents, to seek medical or legal counseling *without parental consent,* even when it is in the best interests of the child." This statement illustrates the committee's intent to undermine the authority of parents, especially those who hold traditional religious beliefs or who would disagree with the committee's radical interpretation of the CRC.

> *The U.N. committee . . . [opposes] the freedom of parents to guide the moral education of their children.*

The definition of medical attention and counseling for adolescents is a continuing area of dispute at U.N. conferences, as illustrated in the preparatory commission reports and final conference proceedings for such meetings as the Cairo International Conference on Population and Development (ICPD) in 1994, the Beijing World Conference on Women in 1995, the ICPD+5 conference in 1999, and the Beijing+5 conference in 2000. The counseling for children is likely to include information on abortion and contraceptives, *regardless of parents' guidance.* The latest, most authoritative research published in the *Journal of the American Medical Association* indicates that opposition by parents to contraception for their teenage children is protective and effective in reducing rates of teen pregnancy. At the Beijing+5 conference, the clash between those who wanted to protect parental rights and those who opposed those rights almost scuttled the possibility of a final conference document.

The U.N. committee's opposition to the freedom of parents to guide the moral education of their children is made clear in a CRC committee rebuke directed at the United Kingdom in 1995. The committee stated that

> insufficient attention has been given to the right of the child to express his/her opinion, including in cases where parents in England and Wales have the possibility of withdrawing their children from parts of the sex education programs in school. In this as in other decisions, including exclusion from school, the child is not systematically invited to express his/her opinion and those opinions may not be given due weight, as required under article 12 of the Convention.

The U.N. committee went even further in its recommendation to the Ethiopian government, urging it to change its laws so that "the limitation of the right to legal counsel of children be abolished as a matter of priority."

Access to Medical Services Without Parental Consent

Consider how direct the CRC committee is in its advice to Austria to increase children's rights over parents' authority: "Austrian Law and regulations do not provide a legal minimum age for medical counseling and treatment *without parental consent* . . . [and] that the requirement of a referral to the courts will dissuade children from seeking medical attention and be prejudicial to the best interests of the child." Austria, like all nations, has defined the age at which the child becomes legally independent of the parent. This effort by the U.N. committee to make states define a different age for medical counseling and treatment is targeted specifically at removing parents' control over the moral formation of their children and the parameters of their children's sexual behavior.

The U.N. committee showed little awareness that Mali [West Africa] is among the poorest countries in the world, with 65 percent of its land area either desert or semi-desert. About 10 percent of the population is nomadic, and some 80 percent of the labor force is engaged in farming and fishing. Per capita GDP [gross domestic product] in Mali in 1998 was estimated to be $790. Yet the U.N. suggests that Mali allocate "adequate hu-

man and financial resources, to develop youth-friendly counseling, care and rehabilitation facilities for adolescents that
would be accessible without parental consent, where this is in
the best interests of the child." The preparatory session leading
up to the Beijing 1995 conference illustrates that making
"counseling" and "rehabilitation facilities" accessible is "U.N.-
speak" for giving government agencies and NGOs the right to
guide minor children toward abortion services and counseling
on contraceptives regardless of the wishes of their parents.

Chipping Away at Parental Authority

The overall agenda is to seek changes in the laws of each nation that will weaken the freedom and authority of parents to
direct the moral education and attitudes of their children.
Nowhere is there a suggestion in the CRC reports to signatory
nations that the role of parents should be strengthened, even
though most parents and observers agree that raising children
is becoming increasingly difficult.

> *Making 'counseling' . . . accessible [to youths]
> is 'U.N.-speak' for giving [agencies] . . . the right to
> guide minor children toward abortion services . . .
> regardless of the wishes of their parents.*

The U.N. demonstrated that it is no longer a friend to parents in its deliberate stand at the First United Nations Conference of Ministers Responsible for Youth, which resulted in pro-
mulgation of the U.N. Declaration on Youth in Lisbon [Portugal]
in August 1998. During the deliberations, the U.N. conference
rejected the inclusion of a statement about the role and importance of marriage, parents, and families to the upbringing of
youth. The U.N. stand prompted an objection from the Vatican,
which

> repeatedly sought to introduce the concept of par-
> ent's rights, duties and responsibilities to provide
> appropriate direction and guidance to their youth,
> in a manner consistent with their evolving capac-
> ities, a right enshrined in the most significant in-

ternational documents of this century. . . . Despite our best joint efforts . . . [the declaration] continues to fail to take into account the vital role which parents must play. . . . [T]here is no language currently in the draft Lisbon Declaration as regards marriage and the creation of the family.

As this statement makes clear, the omission from the declaration of a statement about marriage and a parent's vital role in a child's upbringing was not an oversight; it was deliberate. The U.N. agenda is subverting parental authority and the standing of marriage, regardless of the language in the Universal Declaration of Human Rights.

3

Forced Child Labor Is a Human Rights Abuse

Anti-Slavery International and International Confederation of Free Trade Unions

Founded in 1839, Anti-Slavery International is the world's oldest international human rights organization. It campaigns to eliminate slavery everywhere. The International Confederation of Free Trade Unions (ICFTU) helps to defend workers' rights, eradicate forced and child labor, and promote equal rights for women workers.

Child trafficking and forced labor are grievous human rights violations. Around the world youths are taken from their families (often through deception); transported to a new town or country; and forcibly employed as domestic servants, market traders, field workers, camel jockeys (who race camels), and prostitutes. When a child is completely dependent on an employer, as coerced child laborers are, he or she is vulnerable to extreme exploitation. Trafficked youths, some as young as 4 years old, may be subjected to beatings, starvation, 14- to 18-hour workdays, and other inhumane working conditions. Although several human rights organizations and governments have stipulated that children under 12 years old cannot be employed and that those under 18 cannot perform work that jeopardizes their health, safety, or morals, youths across the globe remain forcibly employed in deplorable environments.

Trafficking in human beings is the fastest growing manifestation of forced labour. A study published in 2000, for the

US Centre for the Study of Intelligence, estimated that between 700,000 and two million women and children were trafficked across borders each year globally. In December 2000, the United Nations [UN] sought to address this problem by adopting a Protocol to Prevent, Suppress and Punish Trafficking in Persons, especially Women and Children to supplement the UN Convention against Transnational Organized Crime.

> *[A United Nations] Protocol seeks to prevent . . . trafficking in persons and also to protect and assist victims of trafficking, with full respect to their human rights.*

The Protocol seeks to prevent and combat trafficking in persons and also to protect and assist victims of trafficking, with full respect to their human rights. It includes, in Article 2, the following definition of trafficking:

This definition is very inclusive. Traffickers are all those who facilitate the recruitment, transportation, transfer, harbouring or receipt of persons through means which would include coercion, deception or by taking advantage of the victim's vulnerability in order to exploit them.

Human Trafficking

The Protocol also seeks to offer extra protection to victims of forced labour by stating in Article 3 that, when coercion, deception or the abuse of authority takes place, then it is irrelevant whether the trafficking victim consented to their exploitation or not. Thus, a woman may agree to be a sex worker in Europe, but then on arrival find that her passport is confiscated, she is forced to work 12 hours a day and she is not paid. In this situation she is a victim of trafficking because she has been deceived as to the conditions of work and therefore the fact that she consented to be a sex worker is irrelevant.

The Protocol also states that the recruitment, transportation, transfer, harbouring or receipt of a child (any person under 18) for the purpose of exploitation should always be considered as trafficking. Those migrant workers who have been trafficked or who have not got a regular immigration status are particularly at risk of being subjected to forced labour because they are afraid that if they go to the authorities to make a complaint or to seek protection they will be deported.

However, even migrants who enter another country with the proper documentation are still at risk of being subjected to forced labour. Migrant domestic workers are particularly vulnerable to forced labour because the nature of their work means that they are invisible to the wider society. Employers may seek to further isolate their domestics by preventing them from leaving the house where they live and work unless they are accompanied, and by confiscating their passport or other identity documents.

Trafficking and Forced Child Labour in Gabon

In 1999, an organisation in Benin [West Africa], *Enfants Solidaires d'Afrique et du Monde* (ESAM), completed a report on the trafficking of children between the Republic of Benin and Gabon. The research was based on interviews with parents, children, receiving families, traffickers and officials. The report found that out of a sample of 229 children who had been trafficked, 86 per cent were girls. This reflects the fact that girls are in greater demand for work as domestics and as market traders. Of the trafficked boys interviewed, most worked in the agricultural or fishing sectors. More than one-third of parents said that they were prepared to hand their children over to traffickers because they could not earn enough to meet the essential needs of their family.

> *The recruitment, transportation, transfer, harbouring or receipt of a child . . . for the purpose of exploitation should always be considered as trafficking.*

A total of 91 children were interviewed in Benin about the conditions in which they lived and worked while they were in Gabon. With regard to their living conditions, more than two-thirds described their treatment as 'bad'. They described being shouted at, being deprived of food and being beaten by their employer as examples of the bad treatment they endured.

With regard to their working conditions, more than half described their treatment as very bad. These children were generally working for traders and had to work between 14 and 18 hours a day—this includes both domestic work and commercial activities. They had to carry heavy loads and walk long distances in order to sell goods.

> *" More than two-thirds [of trafficked children] described their treatment as 'bad'. They described being shouted at, being deprived of food and being beaten by their employer. "*

If the girls did not earn enough money they risked being beaten. This meant that they were often frightened about going home if their earnings for the day were low or if they had been stolen. This makes the girls vulnerable to exploitation by people who offer to pay the money they must give to their employers (who are called "aunties"). However, instead of helping them these men often sexually abuse them or force them into prostitution. The following testimonies taken from different girls after their return to Benin illustrate these dangers:

> "One day, I was coming back from the market crying because a gang had beaten me up and taken all the money I'd made from selling iced juice. A man proposed to give me the money I must give to my auntie but I had to stay with him for a while before returning home. He abused me sexually. He always wants the same thing. Another day, he paid for the whole tray of fruits I was selling, and I had to do the very same thing. I fled from my auntie and found refuge with a Gabonese woman."

> [Another girl said:] "I couldn't sell of lot of fruit that day. I went back home and my auntie beat me because I didn't bring enough money. I ran away to cry behind the house. A man proposed that I spend that night with him and he would pay my auntie the money I owe. The following day, he brought me to a station where we took a bus for Equatorial Guinea [western Africa]. I worked a lot on a planta-

tion and also acted as his wife. One day, I fled by going through the forest until Libreville [Gabon]. From there I was brought back to Benin.". . .

Child Labour Laws

Several international standards identify conditions and circumstances in which no child can be employed. Article 26 of the Universal Declaration of Human Rights stipulates that *"Elementary education shall be compulsory"* thereby prohibiting any work which prevents a child from attending or completing elementary education.

Article 10 of the Economic, Social and Cultural Rights Covenant calls on states to specify a minimum age below which *"the paid employment of children should be prohibited and punishable by law"*.

The ILO [International Labour Organisation] Minimum Age Convention of 1973 (No. 138), provides the only comprehensive set of guidelines relating to the appropriate age at which young children can enter the work force. It also takes into consideration the fact that in less developed countries many families rely on money earned by their children.

ILO Convention No. 138 sets the minimum age for work at not less than the age for finishing compulsory schooling and in any case, not less than 15 years old (14 in countries where the *"economy and educational facilities are insufficiently developed"*). Light work can be done by children between the ages of 13 and 15 years old (reduced to 12 in developing countries), but the Convention does not allow children under 12 to be employed in any circumstances. The minimum age for hazardous work likely to jeopardise the health, safety, or morals of a worker is set at 18 years old.

> *The minimum age for hazardous work likely to jeopardise the health, safety, or morals of a worker is set at 18 years old.*

Article 32 of the UN Convention on the Rights of the Child (1989) calls on governments to ensure that children do not perform *"any work that is likely to be hazardous or to interfere with the child's education or to be harmful to the child's health or physical, mental, spiritual, moral or social development".*

The ILO Bureau of Statistics has estimated that there are 250 million working children between the ages of five and 14 in the world, with some 120 million children working full-time. Many of these children will be working in contravention of the international standards outline above. However, this is in itself does not mean that they are involved in forced child labour.

Forced Child Labour

The general prohibitions on forced labour that have already been discussed apply equality to children. However, additional factors have to be considered when assessing whether a case of child labour can be described as forced labour.

> **"** *In Haiti, children are given away or sold by their parents . . . to work as domestic servants. . . . [The] child is not viewed as a person, but rather as a transferable resource.* **"**

When children are sent to work away from their families, sometimes to a different country, they are made dependent on their employer for their well-being and basic necessities. The child cannot leave because they do not have any money; are too young to find their way home (particularly if they are abroad and do not speak the local language); or are too afraid of what their employers might do to them if they tried to run away. Children are often sent to work in other households or to relatives by their parents because they are having difficulty looking after them or think that their child will be better off working in a more affluent house. This practice particularly affects girls who are then employed as live-in domestics.

Parents are frequently promised that their child will go to school or get job training. Wages are sometimes paid to the parents in advance, particularly if the child has to live some distance from home. In other cases the child receives no wages and works solely for their upkeep.

The complete dependence of the child on their employer means that they are vulnerable to extreme exploitation and

34

abuse. For this reason Article 1(d) of the 1956 Supplementary
Convention specifically prohibits:

> "any institution or practice whereby a child or
> young person under the age of 18 years, is delivered
> by either or both of his natural parents or by his
> guardian to another person, whether for reward or
> not, with a view to the exploitation of the child or
> young person or of his labour".

This type of practice, which often involves coercion, abduction, deception, or the abuse of power or a position of vulnerability, comes under the definition of trafficking as set out in the UN Protocol to Prevent, Suppress and Punish Trafficking in Persons. The Protocol prohibits the trafficking of children for whatever purpose.

The ILO uses Convention No. 29 on forced labour to examine cases of bonded child labour, child sexual exploitation and child domestic work in conditions which are similar to slavery.

Restaveks in Haiti

In Haiti, children are given away or sold by their parents to other families to work as domestic servants. These children are known as *restaveks* and the majority are girls from poor rural backgrounds. The *restaveks* are placed with their employers through an intermediary and contact between the child and their parents is severed, leaving the child completely dependent on her employing family and vulnerable to exploitation.

> *In many cases [child domestic servants] ended up 'preferring a life without shelter or food to a life of servitude and abuse'.*

The *restaveks* child is not viewed as a person, but rather as a transferable resource. If members of the employing family decide at any time that they are not happy with the child, they can throw them out. Yet if the child is unhappy or becomes the victim of abuse they cannot leave. Those who try to run away may be recaptured, beaten and returned to the employing family.

In 1993, the ILO's Committee of Experts reviewed the situation of *restaveks* children under ILO Convention No. 29. The Committee of Experts highlighted three aspects of the situation faced by *restaveks* children which were characteristic of forced labour:

The children's separation from their families;

The fact that the children are not consulted regarding their willingness to work as domestics;

The children's total dependence upon their employing family for their welfare and their consequent vulnerability to extreme exploitation, abuse and other forms of punishment.

> *A four-year-old camel jockey from Bangladesh . . . was found abandoned and close to death in the [United Arab Emirates] desert.*

The Committee commented that *restaveks* children were found ". . . to work as domestics in conditions which are not unlike servitude. The children were forced to work long hours with little chance of bettering their conditions; many children were reported to have been physically and sexually abused".

The Committee of Experts also noted that for many their only choice was to run away and that in many cases they ended up "preferring a life without shelter or food to a life of servitude and abuse. The practice of *restaveks* was openly compared to slavery in Haiti". In 1999, ILO/IPEC estimated between 110,000 and 250,000 children work as *restaveks* in Haiti.

The Worst Forms of Child Labour

In recent years, the ILO has intensified its efforts to eradicate the use of forced child labour internationally. In 1992, the ILO set up the International Programme on the elimination of Child Labour (IPEC) to assist countries in developing and implementing policies and programmes to eliminate child labour. IPEC made the elimination of forced child labour and child bonded labour one of its three priority areas.

In June 1998, the ILO's International Labour Conference adopted the Declaration on Fundamental Principles and Rights at Work, which made the effective abolition of child labour one of its four fundamental principles.

This means that all member states are required to promote the abolition of child labour even if they have not ratified the relevant "core" standard in relation to child labour. These standards are the ILO Minimum Age Convention (No. 138) and the new ILO Convention on the Worst Forms of Child Labour (No. 182) which was adopted in 1999.

The Worst Forms of Child Labour Convention calls on states to take immediate and urgent action to prohibit and eliminate the most abusive and hazardous forms of exploitation, now referred to as the "worst forms" of child labour. The definition of "the worst forms of child labour" is presented in Article 3 and includes:

> (a) all forms of slavery or practices similar to slavery such as the sale and trafficking of children, debt bondage and serfdom and forced or compulsory labour, including the forced or compulsory recruitment of children for use in armed conflict.

The accompanying recommendation proposes that governments establish programmes of action to identify the forms of child labour which require elimination and then to take the necessary measures to effectively abolish them.

Forced Child Labour in the United Arab Emirates

Very young children from the Indian sub-continent and various parts of Africa have been kidnapped or trafficked to the United Arab Emirates (UAE) to work as camel jockeys [i.e., they race camels].

The fact that children are separated from their families, taken to a country where the people, culture and usually the language are completely unknown and left completely dependent on their employers for their very survival means that they are not in a position to stop working and are vulnerable to extreme exploitation and physical abuse.

Despite the fact that Article 20 of the UAE's 1980 labour legislation prohibits the employment of anyone under the age of 15, the UN Special Rapporteur on the sale of children noted in her 1999 report that little was being done to stop the use of underage children as camel jockeys. She found evidence that:

". . . clearly indicates that the rules are being blatantly ignored. In February 1998, ten Bangladeshi boys, aged between five and eight, were rescued in India while being smuggled to become camel jockeys. The boys had been lured away from their poor families with the promise of high-paying jobs".

During 1999 and 2000, a number of cases involving the trafficking or abuse of camel jockeys were reported. One involved a four-year-old camel jockey from Bangladesh who was found abandoned and close to death in the UAE desert. In a separate case another four-year-old from Bangladesh had his legs severely burnt by his employer as a punishment for "under performing".

4

Sweatshops Benefit Children

Radley Balko

Radley Balko, a freelance writer and policy analyst with the Cato Institute, has published articles on issues ranging from free trade to drug prohibition.

Sweatshops are factories whose working conditions would horrify most westerners. However, in third world countries, where poverty dictates that every family member must work to survive, sweatshops provide needed employment for many children. In fact, when Western countries boycott or close factories in an attempt to protest their employment practices, children are the most adversely affected. In the absence of sweatshops, youths must earn money in much more dangerous and exploitative positions, such as prostitution. Rather than push for boycotts of goods made in sweatshops, the United States must allow the sweatshops to continue competing with each other for employees. This will gradually lead to an increase in workers' wages and, in turn, a prospering economy. Ultimately, a flourishing economy will benefit children and will eventually enable third world countries to ban child labor.

Two reporters relay this anecdote from Thailand:

> One of the half-dozen men and women sitting on a bench eating was a sinewy, bare-chested laborer in his late 30's named Mongkol Latlakorn. It was a hot, lazy day, and so we started chatting idly about the food and, eventually, our families. Mongkol

mentioned that his daughter, Darin, was 15, and his voice softened as he spoke of her. She was beautiful and smart, and her father's hopes rested on her.

"Is she in school?" we asked.

"Oh, no," Mongkol said, his eyes sparkling with amusement. "She's working in a factory in Bangkok [Thailand]. She's making clothing for export to America." He explained that she was paid $2 a day for a nine-hour shift, six days a week.

"It's dangerous work," Mongkol added. "Twice the needles went right through her hands. But the managers bandaged up her hands, and both times she got better again and went back to work."

"How terrible," we murmured sympathetically.

So begins Nicholas Kristof and Sheryl WuDunn's article on sweatshops for the *New York Times* a few years ago [in 2000]. The two had lived off and on in Asia for 14 years, and were researching their upcoming book on emerging Asian economies, *Thunder From the East*. Like most westerners, Kristof and WuDunn arrived in Asia horrified by the sweatshop conditions they'd heard about and witnessed. Like most westerners—accustomed to 40-max hour workweeks, sick leave, and vacation—the two were outraged at the way western companies exploited third world labor. But read on:

Mongkol looked up, puzzled. "It's good pay," he said. "I hope she can keep that job. There's all this talk about factories closing now, and she said there are rumors that her factory might close. I hope that doesn't happen. I don't know what she would do then."

Mongkol's story illustrates how, by the time they wrote their book, Kristof and WuDunn had significantly upgraded their opinion of sweatshops. While regrettable, they concluded, sweatshops are a crucial and necessary step in most economies' evolution to prosperity.

Kristoff and WuDunn are right, of course. And efforts to ban, boycott, or otherwise shut down third world factories bring nothing but harm to the people they employ. Removing the best of a handful of bad options doesn't benefit the poor at all. It hurts them. And sometimes it kills them. Examples abound:

• In the early 1990s, the United States Congress considered the "Child Labor Deterrence Act," which would have taken punitive action against companies benefiting from child labor. The Act never passed, but the public debate it triggered put enormous pressure on a number of multinational corporations with assets in the U.S. One German garment maker laid off 50,000 child workers in Bangladesh. The British charity organization Oxfam later conducted a study that found that thousands of those laid-off children later became prostitutes, turned to crime, or starved to death.

> *Thousands of . . . laid-off children later became prostitutes, turned to crime, or starved to death.*

• The United Nations organization UNICEF reports that an international boycott of the Nepalese carpet industry in the mid-1990s caused several plants to shut down; thousands of Nepalese girls later entered the sex trade.

• In 1995, a consortium of anti-sweatshop groups threw the spotlight on football (soccer) stitching plants in Pakistan. In response, Nike and Reebok shut down their plants in Pakistan, and several other companies followed suit. The result: tens of thousands of unemployed Pakistanis. Mean income in Pakistan fell by 20%. According to University of Colorado economist Keith E. Maskus, studies later showed a large proportion of those laid off ended up in crime, begging, or working as prostitutes.

• In 2000 the BBC did an expose on sweatshop factories in Cambodia with ties to both Nike and the Gap. The BBC uncovered unsavory working conditions, and found several examples of children under 15 years of age working 12 or more hour shifts. After the BBC expose aired, both Nike and the Gap pulled out of Cambodia under public pressure. Cambodia lost $10 million in contracts, and hundreds of Cambodians lost their jobs.

Third World Countries Need the Advantage of Cheap Labor

In truth, every prosperous country on the planet today went through an industrial period heavily reliant on sweatshop labor. The United States, Britain, France, Sweden and others all rode to modernity on the backs of child laborers. The choice was simple: kids worked, or they went hungry. It wasn't a terribly rosy set of choices, but at least the choice was available. Anti-globalization activists are doing their damndest to make sure choice *isn't* available to those living in today's fledgling economies.

Critics counter that unlike in the early 20th century, western companies today are wealthy enough to pay "living" wages, to establish comfortable working conditions, and to protect third world environments. They may be right.

But then, what advantage would there be to investing in the developing world in the first place? Cheap labor is the only chit the third world has to lure much-needed western investment. Take it away, and there's no reason for western corporations to incur the costs of putting up factories, shipping, security and the bevy of other expenses that come with maintaining plants overseas.

One of free trade's chief critics admits as much. In the introduction to his book *The Race to the Bottom*, anti-globalization icon Alan Tonelson writes the following, in reference to the World Trade Organization:

> Most of the organization's third world members— or at least their governments—opposed including any labor rights and environmental protections in trade agreements. They viewed low wages and lax pollution control laws as major assets they could offer to international investors—prime lures for job-creating factories and the capital they so desperately needed for other development-related purposes. Indeed, they observed, most rich countries ignored the environment and limited workers' power (to put it kindly) early in their economic histories. Why should today's developing countries be held to higher standards?

Tonelson, of course, was on his way to making another point. But he inadvertently revealed an inconsistency that will always plague the legitimacy of anti-globalist logic: boycotts, "fair trade" regulations and public pressure do nothing to punish the corporations who benefit from sweatshops. They punish only third world laborers and, to a lesser extent, western consumers.

How Free Trade Beats Sweatshops

The best way to lessen the plight of sweatshop workers is more free trade, not less. If workers make 75 cents per day in factory A—the only plant in town—the best thing that could happen to them would be for a second factory to open up. If Factory B pays less than 75 cents, it won't attract any workers. If it offers exactly 75 cents, it might attract a few workers who couldn't get jobs at factory A. If it pays more than 75 cents, however, it might attract the best and brightest from factory A. Factory A then must decide whether to up its wages, or look for new labor—which means more jobs.

> " The United States, Britain, France, Sweden and others all rode to modernity on the backs of child laborers. "

The alternative: force factory A to pay artificially high wages. That negates the advantage factory A had by investing in a developing country in the first place. Factory A packs up and returns to the U.S. Factory B never happens, because factory B's parent company sees no advantage (see: cheap labor) in investing in the developing country. Factory A's workers' wages go from 75 cents per day to nothing.

Instead of two factories paying twice as many workers higher wages, enabling them to inch their way out of poverty, a community is left with no factories, no jobs, and no hope.

Sweatshops Lead to Success

Recent history teems with examples of how sweatshop labor has helped poor economies leap to prosperity. And given the interconnectivity and technology available in the current world economy—and that there's lots of western wealth to help them along—they can make the leap in a fraction of the time it took the west.

Kristoff and WuDunn note, for example, that it took Britain 58 years to double per capita GDP [gross domestic product] after its industrial revolution. China—home to millions of sweatshop workers—doubles its per capita GDP every ten years. In the sweatshop-dotted southern providence of Dongguan, wages have increased fivefold in just the last few years. "A private housing market has appeared," Kristof and WuDunn write, "and video arcades and computer schools have opened to cater to workers with rising incomes . . . a hint of a middle class has appeared."

If China's provinces were separate countries, the two authors write, the 20 fastest growing economies from 1978 to 1995 would all have been Chinese.

Swedish economist Johan Norberg writes in his book *In Defense of Global Capitalism* that where it took Sweden 80 years to reach modernity, it has taken Taiwan and Hong Kong just 25. He predicts that all of South and East Asia will be prosperous enough to ban child labor entirely by 2010.

But that's just it. A country must be able to *afford* to ban child labor before child labor is pulled out from under it. Otherwise, without work, the children there beg, or starve, or die of malaria, or diarrhea.

China, Taiwan, Hong Kong—all accepted sweatshop labor as an unsavory stepping stone to prosperity.

Contrast those nations to the countries that have traditionally been "spared" sweatshops: the results are striking.

India, for example, has long resisted allowing itself to be "exploited" by foreign investment. It was one of the last major countries in the world to be introduced to Coca-Cola. Consequently, India festered in abject poverty for decades. India has only opened its markets to the west in the latter part of the last century and, as Norberg writes, its economy immediately showed signs of life. India's percentage of child laborers in the workforce has fallen from 35% to just 12%.

5

Minors Should Have the Right to Consent to an Abortion

Planned Parenthood Federation of America

Affiliates of Planned Parenthood Federation of America, the world's largest voluntary family planning organization, provide medical services and sex education to millions of women, men, and teenagers.

Some pregnant teens cannot tell their parents about their pregnancy or planned abortion for fear of abuse. As a result, most states recognize youths' right to consent to their own reproductive health care. However, the proposed Child Custody Protection Act (CCPA) would make it a federal crime for a minor's family or friends to help her receive an abortion without her parents' approval, which raises serious implications for adolescents' rights. Besides subjecting to penalties the very people who can assist teens in their time of need, the bill would eliminate confidentiality from youths' health care. Furthermore, the CCPA's parental consent process is difficult and time-consuming, thereby delaying a girl's abortion. This delay threatens teens' health, as a later abortion is a more dangerous one.

Of all the abortion-related policy issues facing decision-makers in this country today, parental consent or notification before a minor may obtain an abortion is one of the most difficult. Few would deny that most teenagers, especially younger ones, would benefit from adult guidance when faced with an un-

44

wanted pregnancy. Few would deny that such guidance ideally should come from the teenager's parents. Unfortunately, we do not live in an ideal world. For a variety of reasons, including fear of parental maltreatment or abuse, teenagers frequently cannot tell their parents about their pregnancies or planned abortions.

> *[Due to] fear of paternal maltreatment or abuse, teenagers frequently cannot tell their parents about their pregnancies or planned abortions.*

In the 34 states with laws in effect that mandate the involvement of at least one parent in the abortion decision, teenagers who cannot tell their parents must either travel out of state or obtain approval from a judge—known as a "judicial bypass" procedure—to obtain an abortion. The result is almost always a delay that can increase both the cost of the abortion and the physical and emotional health risk to the teenager, since an earlier abortion is a safer one.

Currently, anti-choice members of Congress are seeking to make it even more difficult for minors living in states with mandatory parental involvement laws to obtain an abortion with the so-called "Child Custody Protection Act" (CCPA). The bill would make it a federal crime to transport a minor across state lines for an abortion unless the parental involvement requirements of her home state had been met. If the bill were enacted, persons convicted would be subject to imprisonment, fines, and civil suits.[1]

Requiring Parental Consent for Abortion Is Not Consistent with State Laws

Proponents of mandated parental involvement contend that parents have a right to decide what medical services their minor children receive. However, states have long recognized that many minors have the capacity to consent to their own medical care and that, in certain critical areas such as mental health, drug and/or alcohol addiction, treatment for sexually

---

1. As of early 2005, the Child Custody Protection Act had passed in the House but not in the Senate.

transmitted infections (STIs), and pregnancy, entitlement to confidential care is a public health necessity.

• Twenty-one states and the District of Columbia grant all minors the authority to consent to contraceptive services. Approximately eleven other states grant most minors this authority.

• Thirty-four states and the District of Columbia authorize a pregnant minor to obtain prenatal care and delivery services without parental consent or notification.

• All 50 states and the District of Columbia give minors the authority to consent to the diagnosis and treatment of sexually transmitted infections.

Many of these laws allow minors to give consent to treatments that involve greater medical risk than a first-trimester abortion, such as surgical interventions during pregnancy and cesarean sections. Nevertheless, many of these same states require parental consent for abortion.

Many Teens Have Compelling Reasons to Seek Confidential Services

A minority of teenagers do not involve their parents. Overwhelmingly, they make this decision for compelling reasons. A 1991 study of unmarried minors having abortions in states without parental involvement laws found that

• Sixty-one percent of the respondents reported that at least one of their parents knew about their abortion.

• Of those minors who did not inform their parents of their abortions, 30 percent had histories of violence in their families, feared the occurrence of violence, or were afraid of being forced to leave their homes.

• Minors who did not tell their parents were also disproportionately older (aged 16 or 17) and employed.

• Among the respondents who did not inform their parents of their pregnancies, all consulted someone in addition to clinic staff about their abortions, such as their boyfriend (89 percent), an adult (52 percent), or a professional (22 percent).

Lack of Confidential Reproductive Health Care Harms Teenagers

Evidence suggests that lack of confidentiality in accessing sexual health care services severely delays or even curtails minors' use of those services. A survey of abortion patients around the U.S., conducted by the Alan Guttmacher Institute (AGI), found that 63% of minors who were having later abortions (after 16 weeks' gestation) cited fear of telling their parents as reason for the delay. In August 2002, the *Journal of the American Medical Association* published a study of minors seeking sexual health care services at Planned Parenthood health centers in Wisconsin. Nearly half (47%) of the respondents reported that they would discontinue use of all Planned Parenthood services if their parents were notified that they were seeking prescription contraceptives. An additional 12% would delay or discontinue using specific sexual health care services if parental notification were required. But only one percent said they would stop having vaginal intercourse.

> *Minors have the capacity to consent to their own medical care and . . . [in the area of] pregnancy, entitlement to confidential care is a public health necessity.*

Experience shows that teenagers who cannot involve their parents in their abortion services suffer harm in states with mandatory parental consent and notice laws. Whether they travel to other states or obtain judicial approval, the results are the same: delays that can greatly increase both the physical and emotional health risks as well as the costs.

• While nationwide most minors seeking judicial approval receive it, the process is unwieldy and, most importantly, time-consuming. Court proceedings in Minnesota routinely delayed abortions by more than one week, and sometimes up to three weeks.

• In Minnesota, the proportion of second-trimester abortions among minors terminating their pregnancies increased by 18 percent following enactment of a parental notification law. Likewise, since Missouri's parental consent law went into effect in 1985, the proportion of second-trimester abortions among minors increased from 19 percent in 1985 to 23 percent in 1988.

• Studies conducted in Pennsylvania and Alabama found that the vast majority of courts in those states were unprepared to implement the judicial bypass. Some court officials had not even heard of the laws, despite the fact that they had been in effect for several years.

• The manner in which each state enforces its judicial bypass laws is erratic. In Minnesota, the federal district court found that the state courts "denied only an infinitesimal proportion of the petitions brought since 1981," [according to the American Civil Liberties Union]. A study in Massachusetts found that only nine of the 477 abortion requests studied had been denied. However, an Ohio report found that the percentage of waivers denied ranged from 100 percent to 2 percent, depending on the county in which the petition was filed.

Compliance with the Law Is Difficult

Some states go as far as to require the involvement of both parents. These statutes ignore the realities of teenagers' lives.

• In 2000, approximately 19 million children under the age of 18 lived with only one parent. Nearly three million more lived with neither parent.

• In 2000, 33 percent of all births occurred to unmarried women. One study found that 20 percent of unmarried fathers had little to no contact with their children.

• Millions of children live with a single parent subsequent to divorce. In 2000, 54 percent of single parents with children under the age of 18 were divorced or separated. A study found that one-third of divorced fathers had no contact with their children during the previous year.

> Lack of confidentiality in accessing sexual health care services severely delays or even curtails minors' use of those services.

• In Minnesota, more than one-quarter of the teenagers who sought judicial bypass were accompanied by one parent, who was most often divorced or separated. According to the federal district court that reviewed Minnesota's law [in *Hodgson v. Minnesota*], many of the custodial parents feared that notification would "bring the absent parent back into the family in an intrusive and abusive way."

Moreover, even if a teenager is able and willing to involve

one or both parents, the procedures required by some state parental consent or notification laws make compliance impossible or difficult.

• Requiring that teenagers either obtain notarized evidence that parents have been notified or present a death certificate for a deceased parent may present impossible logistical barriers, lead to breaches of confidentiality for parents and teenagers, or cause serious delay.

> ❝ Some states go as far as to require the involvement of both parents [in a minor's abortion]. These statutes ignore the realities of teenagers' lives. ❞

• A requirement that the physician personally locate and notify the parents could easily both delay the procedure and increase the cost.

The Child Custody Protection Act Harms Minors

In April 2003, the CCPA was reintroduced in the House of Representatives and the Senate. The bill would make it a federal crime to transport a minor across state lines to obtain abortion services without fulfilling the parental consent or notice requirements of her home state. In 1998, the House of Representatives passed the bill by a vote of 276 to 150, but President [Bill] Clinton threatened to veto it, and the Senate never took it up for consideration. In 1999, the House Judiciary Committee passed the CCPA, defeating five proposed amendments, including those that would create exceptions for grandparents, siblings, aunts and uncles, and clergy who assist minors in obtaining abortions. That year, the legislation passed in the full House of Representatives again, this time by a vote of 270 to 159. However, the Senate again failed to take it up for consideration. Although, if passed, the Act would only affect a small percentage of women seeking abortion services—minors account for fewer than one in 10 abortions performed—the impact of the Act would be dramatic.

• The CCPA would subject to criminal penalties anyone—a

grandparent, adult sibling, member of the clergy, or medical professional—who assists a minor in traveling across state lines to receive an abortion without the parental consent or notification required by her home state.

• CCPA makes such assistance a crime even if confidential abortions are legal in the state where the abortion is to be performed and even if that state allows the accompanying grandparent or adult sibling to give lawful consent for the minor's abortion.

• CCPA thus isolates young women from the trusted friends and relatives who can assist them in time of crisis.

• The CCPA makes criminals out of family members and friends even in emergency situations when the minor needs an immediate abortion to protect her health.

• The CCPA potentially requires a minor to satisfy differing legal requirements in two states: the state she comes from and the state where she is to have the abortion. If those two states both have parental consent or notice requirements, the minor may have to seek waivers from judges in two states, further delaying her abortion and raising its costs and health risks.

• Because 87% of U.S. counties lack an abortion provider, CCPA will increase the burdens on the many young women who must cross state lines simply to access the nearest abortion provider.

• The CCPA also raises a number of other constitutional and legal questions, particularly those related to issues of federalism. The legislation effectively nullifies the laws of those states that allow physicians to provide confidential services to minors who enter the states for abortion and deprives individuals of their right to cross state lines to obtain lawful services. Such intervention by the federal government would be unprecedented, and raises serious implications for states, and individuals' rights.

6

Abortion Violates a Child's Rights

Scott Tibbs

Scott Tibbs cofounded the Hoosier Review, *a conservative alternative to Indiana University–Bloomington's newspaper, to distribute political news and commentary about campus, state, and international issues.*

An unborn child has the right to be physically and legally shielded from harm. This includes protection from abortion, the brutal killing of fetuses by their mothers. Because the Fourteenth Amendment guarantees equal protection for all, homicide laws must safeguard the unborn just like every other person. Never should a woman's right to privacy and personal autonomy supersede the unborn child's right to live. Even if a woman has been forcibly impregnated by a rapist, she does not have the right to kill her baby. Nor should a mother be permitted to abort simply because her fetus is determined to have a severe deformity; that would be just as wrong as killing the sick or the elderly. Fetuses at all stages of development are humans, and all humans have a right to life.

January 22nd, 2003 marks the 30th anniversary of *Roe v. Wade,* the Supreme Court decision that declared women have a "constitutional right" to kill their unborn children. Norma McCorvey, the "Jane Roe" in that case, is now a pro-life activist. Since that decision, over 42 million unborn babies have died at the hands of America's lucrative abortion industry. This number dwarfs the number of people killed in the Nazi Holocaust. As we approach this anniversary of shame, it is reasonable to review why abortion should be prohibited.

Let's look at the facts. When sperm and egg cells meet, a new life is created. The embryo has a completely new DNA code, separate from any other being in the world. All of the building blocks necessary for that new life to grow and develop are present at fertilization. The only thing added from that point forward is nutrition, shelter, and time. Any biology text-book can confirm this fact.

Protections Begin at Fertilization

The next question is when should life be protected? Opinions vary widely on this. Princeton University professor Peter Singer, known as the "father of the animal rights movement", argues that a baby does not have a right to life even after birth, and that infanticide is morally acceptable. Some pro-abortion extremists won't go as far as Singer, but do advocate that birth be the dividing line. They argue that a woman's right to per-sonal autonomy over her body is paramount over the right to life of the unborn child growing inside her. But does personal autonomy justify killing?

The answer is no. No one should be in the position of de-ciding whether another human being lives or dies. Pregnancy is part of a natural biological process. The fetus is not a parasite using the mother's body against her will; it is part of the process that perpetuates the human race. Each human being has an intrinsic worth and a moral right to life.

> *The fetus is not a parasite using the mother's body against her will; it is part of the process that perpetuates the human race.*

The *Herald-Times* ran a staff editorial on January 19th [2002] noting that most people remain somewhere in the mid-dle on abortion. Outside of the 40% that say abortion should either always be legal or always be illegal, 59% say it should be legal "sometimes". Even in that group, opinions vary wildly on what "sometimes" means.

If the unborn are offered some sort of legal protection,

when should that protection begin? Should it be at a heartbeat, or when brainwaves can be first detected, or when the baby is sufficiently developed to feel pain? What about a specific time frame like the first trimester?

> *If one truly believes that an unborn child deserves a right to life, the circumstances of his or her conception should not invalidate this right.*

The only logical place to begin protection of the unborn is at fertilization. This is the point where a new human being is created. The problem with using a specific point in the stage of a baby's development as where he or she deserved protection is that it is arbitrary. If a baby cannot be killed once we can detect a heartbeat or brain waves, then what is so different two days earlier? What is so special about these specific points in development? Prohibiting abortions at specific times (only allowing abortions in the first trimester, for example) is even more arbitrary. Protecting the unborn from fertilization onward is the most consistent way of approaching a pro-life viewpoint.

No Exceptions

Even many people who call themselves "pro-life" begin to weaken when asked about the hard cases: rape, incest, and severe fetal deformity. But should a ban on abortion make room for these exceptions?

If one believes that the unborn child is a human being, deserving of protection from direct, intentional harm, why is the situation different in the case of rape and incest? Is the unborn baby any less human? If not, then why should an unborn baby be punished for the sins of his or her father? Some would say that a rape victim has been through enough, and should not be forced to carry a rapist's baby to term. But does one crime of violence justify another? No. If one truly believes that an unborn child deserves a right to life, the circumstances of his or her conception should not invalidate this right. Either an unborn baby is worthy of protection or not. Unfortunately, many "pro-life" politicians allow for this exception only because they fear being labeled "extreme", which could cost them votes.

What about severe fetal deformity? A true pro-life position would not allow for this exception either. No one has the right to make a decision on who would have a sufficiently low "quality of life" to justify killing him or her. Just as most people balk at killing the elderly or infirm without their consent, we should recoil at the thought of killing an unborn child because of our own judgments that he or she would not be "happy" if given a chance to live.

Murder and the Right to Privacy

Many will argue that this is a women's issue, and that men should not have a right to make a decision in the matter. (Of course, usually when one reads or hears this argument, it is in regard to why a man should not be able to advocate restrictions on or prohibition of abortion. The opinions of pro-"choice" men are okay.) This is a classic example of the *ad hominem* logical fallacy. Why is an argument that may be valid when made by a female suddenly not valid when a man makes the exact same argument? The logical merits of whether or not abortion should be prohibited do not change regardless of who is making that argument, whether it is a man, a woman, or a five-eyed space alien from Mars.

> *Allowing abortion violates the 14th Amendment by denying the unborn equal protection under homicide laws.*

Roe itself is quite flawed. The Supreme Court sidestepped the question of fetal personhood and declared that an implied "right to privacy" in the Constitution made prohibitions on abortion unconstitutional. But one cannot make a legal decision on abortion without considering personhood. Indeed, the 14th Amendment declares that "nor shall any State . . . deny to any person within its jurisdiction the equal protection of the laws". Allowing abortion violates the 14th Amendment by denying the unborn equal protection under homicide laws.

In addition, the Constitution does not contain an absolute "right to privacy". The Fourth Amendment guarantees that the people will not be subject to "unreasonable" searches and seizures. But government reserves the right to search someone's home, papers and possessions if the proper legal channels are filed. In any case, a "right to privacy" certainly does not include the right to kill another human being.

Even while pro-lifers want to eliminate abortion altogether, even those who hold the most extreme pro-abortion positions often say the number of abortions is way too high. Former President Bill Clinton, whose pro-abortion views are so extreme that he twice vetoed a ban on the heinous procedure known as "partial-birth abortion", has said that he wants abortion to be "safe, legal, and *rare*." Clearly, the status quo is not acceptable. While the number of abortions has decreased in recent years, the figure of 1.2 million babies killed per year is still astronomically high. That amounts to an average of 3,287 abortions every single day. As *Roe v. Wade* enters its fourth decade, and after 42 million babies [have been] brutally killed, isn't it time to say, "enough is enough"?

7

Students' Rights Are Too Far-Reaching

Kay S. Hymowitz

Kay S. Hymowitz writes extensively on education and childhood. She is the author of Ready or Not: What Happens When We Treat Small Children as Adults.

The courts and the federal government have granted students too many rights while curtailing educators' power to control youths who exhibit criminal tendencies. In the 1960s and 1970s, court rulings guaranteed students the right to education, free expression, and due process, severely limiting school officials' ability to expel wrongdoers, regulate disruptive speech, and suspend schoolchildren without holding a hearing. Meting out punishments has since become a time-consuming and frustrating process for administrators. Complicating matters, schools are required by federal law to provide education to disabled students and are rarely allowed to punish them for wrongdoing. This becomes especially problematic when the definition of *disabled* is extended to include youths with simple learning problems, whose disruptive or aggressive acts become unpunishable. As witnesses to these events, students come to the dangerous realization that they can challenge school officials, and they lose respect for their teachers.

Ask Americans what worries them most about the public schools, and the answer might surprise you: discipline. For several decades now, poll after poll shows it topping the list of parents' concerns. Recent news stories—from the Columbine

[High School] massacre to [Reverend] Jesse Jackson's protests against the expulsion of six brawling Decatur, Illinois, high school students to the killing of one Flint, Michigan, six-year-old by another—guarantee that the issue won't lose its urgency any time soon.

> *The courts and the federal government have hacked away at the power of educators to maintain a safe and civil school environment.*

Though fortunately only a small percentage of schools will ever experience real violence, the public's sense that something has gone drastically wrong with school discipline isn't mistaken. Over the past 30 years or so, the courts and the federal government have hacked away at the power of educators to maintain a safe and civil school environment. Rigid school bureaucracies and psychobabble-spouting "experts" have twisted such authority as remains into alien—and alienating—shapes, so that kids today are more likely than ever to go to disorderly schools, whose only answers to the disorder are ham-fisted rules and therapeutic techniques designed to manipulate students' behavior, rather than to initiate them into a genuine civil and moral order. What's been lost is educators' crucial role of passing on cultural values to the young and instructing them in how to behave through innumerable small daily lessons and examples. If the children become disruptive and disengaged, who can be surprised?

The Erosion of School Discipline

School discipline today would be a tougher problem than ever, even without all these changes, because of the nationwide increase of troubled families and disorderly kids. Some schools, especially those in inner cities, even have students who are literally violent felons. High school principal Nora Rosensweig of Green Acres, Florida, estimates that she has had 20 to 25 such felons in her school over the last three years [1997–2000], several of them sporting the electronic ankle bracelets that keep track of paroled criminals. "The impact that one of those students has on 100 kids is amazing," Rosensweig observes. Some

58

students, she says, find them frightening. Others, intrigued, see them as rebel heroes.

But today principals lack the tools they used to have for dealing even with the unruliest kids. Formerly, they could expel such kids permanently or send them to special schools for the hard-to-discipline. The special schools have largely vanished, and state education laws usually don't allow for permanent expulsion. So at best a school might manage to transfer a student felon elsewhere in the same district. New York City principals sometimes engage in a black-humored game of exchanging these "Fulbright Scholars," as they jokingly call them: "I'll take two of yours, if you take one of mine, and you'll owe me."

School Officials Are Barred from Properly Punishing Disabled Students

Educators today also find their hands tied when dealing with another disruptive—and much larger—group of pupils, those covered by the 1975 Individuals with Disabilities Education Act (IDEA). This law, which mandates that schools provide a "free and appropriate education" for children regardless of disability—and provide it, moreover, within regular classrooms whenever humanly possible—effectively strips educators of the authority to transfer or to suspend for long periods any student classified as needing special education.

> We have examples of kids who have sexually assaulted their teacher and are then returned to the classroom.

This wouldn't matter if special education included mainly the wheelchair-bound or deaf students whom we ordinarily think of as disabled. But it doesn't. Over the past several decades, the number of children classified under the vaguely defined disability categories of "learning disability" and "emotional disturbance" has exploded. Many of these kids are those once just called "unmanageable" or "antisocial": part of the legal definition of emotional disturbance is "an inability to build or maintain satisfactory interpersonal relationships with peers and teachers"—in other words, to be part of an orderly community. Prosecutors will tell you that disproportionate numbers of the juvenile criminals they now see are special-ed students.

With IDEA restrictions hampering them, school officials can't respond forcefully when these kids get into fights, curse teachers, or even put students and staff at serious risk, as too often happens. One example captures the law's absurdity. School officials in Connecticut caught one student passing a gun to another on school premises. One, a regular student, received a yearlong suspension, as federal law requires. The other, disabled (he stuttered), received just a 45-day suspension and special, individualized services, as IDEA requires. Most times, though, schools can't get even a 45-day respite from the chaos these kids can unleash. "They are free to do things in school that will land them in jail when they graduate," says Bruce Hunter, an official of the American Association of School Administrators. Laments Julie Lewis, staff attorney for the National School Boards Association: "We have examples of kids who have sexually assaulted their teacher and are then returned to the classroom."

Educators Face Obstacles in Regulating Student Speech

Discipline in the schools isn't primarily about expelling sex offenders and kids who pack guns, of course. Most of the time, what's involved is the "get your feet off the table" or "don't whisper in class" kind of discipline that allows teachers to assume that kids will follow the commonplace directions they give hundreds of times daily. Thanks to two Supreme Court decisions of the late 1960s and the 1970s, though, this everyday authority has come under attack, too.

The first decision, *Tinker v. Des Moines School District*, came about in 1969, after a principal suspended five high school students for wearing black armbands in protest against the Vietnam War. *Tinker* found that the school had violated students' free-speech rights. "It can hardly be argued," wrote Justice Abe Fortas for the majority, "that students or teachers shed their constitutional rights to free speech or expression at the schoolhouse gate." Schools cannot be "enclaves of totalitarianism" nor can officials have "absolute authority over their students," the court solemnly concluded.

Quite possibly the principal in *Tinker* made an error in judgment. But by making matters of school discipline a constitutional issue, the court has left educators fumbling their way through everyday disciplinary encounters with kids ever since. "At each elementary and middle school door, you have some guy making a constitutional decision every day," observes Jeff Krausman, legal counsel to several Iowa school districts. Suppose, says Krausman by way of example, that a student shows up at school wearing a T-shirt emblazoned WHITE POWER. The principal wants to send the kid home to change, but he's not sure it's within his authority to do so, so he calls the superintendent. The superintendent is also unsure, so he calls the district's lawyer. The lawyer's concern, though, isn't that the child has breached the boundaries of respect and tolerance, and needs an adult to tell him so, but whether disciplining the student would violate the First Amendment. Is this, in other words, literally a federal case?

> *By making matters of school discipline a constitutional issue, the court has left educators . fumbling their way through everyday disciplinary encounters with kids.*

And that's not easy to answer. "Where do you draw the line?" Krausman asks. "Some lawyers say you should have to prove that something is "significantly disruptive." But in Iowa you might have a hard time proving that a T-shirt saying WHITE POWER or ASIANS ARE GEEKS is significantly disruptive." Meanwhile, educators' power to instill civility and order in school dissolves into tendentious debates over the exact meaning of legal terms like "significantly disruptive."

The Complications Caused by Student Due-Process Rights

In 1975, the Supreme Court hampered school officials' authority yet further in *Goss v. Lopez*, a decision that expanded the due-process rights of students. *Goss* concerned several students suspended for brawling in the school lunchroom. Though the principal who suspended them actually witnessed the fight himself, the court concluded that he had failed to give the students an adequate hearing before lowering the boom. Students, pronounced the court, are citizens with a property right to their education. To deny that right requires, at the least, an informal hearing with notice, witnesses, and the like; suspensions for longer than ten days might require even more formal procedures.

Following *Tinker's* lead, *Goss* brought lawyers and judges deeper inside the schoolhouse. You want to suspend a violent troublemaker? Because of *Goss*, you now had to ask: Would a judge find your procedures satisfactory? Would he agree that you have enough witnesses? The appropriate documentation? To suspend a student became a time-consuming and frustrating business.

Students soon learned that, if a school official does something they don't like, they can sue him, or at least threaten to do so. New York City special-ed teacher Jeffrey Gerstel's story is sadly typical. Last year [1999], Gerstel pulled a student out of his classroom as he was threatening to kill the assistant teacher. The boy collided with a bookcase and cut his back, though not badly enough to need medical attention. Even so, Gerstel found himself at a hearing, facing the student's indignant mother, who wanted to sue, and three "emotionally disturbed adolescents"—classmates of the boy—who witnessed the scuffle. The mother soon settled the dispute out of court and sent her son back to Gerstel's classroom. But by then, Gerstel had lost the confidence that he needed to handle a roomful of volatile teenagers, and the kids knew it. For the rest of the year, they taunted him: "I'm going to get my mother up here and bring you up on charges."

> *Students soon learned that, if a school official does something they don't like, they can sue him, or at least threaten to do so.*

In another typical recent case, a Saint Charles, Missouri, high schooler running for student council handed out condoms as a way of drumming up votes. The school suspended him. He promptly sued on free-speech grounds; in previous student council elections, he whined, candidates had handed out candy. Though he lost his case, his ability to stymie adults in such a matter, even if only temporarily, could not but give him an enlarged sense of his power against the school authorities: his adolescent fantasy of rebellion had come true.

These days, school lawyers will tell you, this problem is clearing up: in recent years, they point out, the courts have usually sided with schools in discipline cases, as they did in Missouri. But the damage done by *Tinker, Goss,* and their ilk isn't so easily undone. Lawsuits are expensive and time-consuming, even if you win. More important, the mere potential for a lawsuit shrinks the adult in the child's eyes. It transforms the person who should be the teacher and the representative of society's moral and cultural values into a civil servant who may or may not please the young, rights-armed citizen. The natural relationship between adult and child begins to crumble.

> *[Lawsuits transform] the person who should be the teacher and the representative of society's moral and cultural values into a civil servant [of] . . . the young, rights-armed citizen.*

The architects of IDEA, *Tinker,* and *Goss,* of course, thought of themselves as progressive reformers, designing fairer, more responsive schools. Introducing the rights of free speech and due process, they imagined, would ensure that school officials would make fewer "arbitrary and capricious" decisions. But lawmakers failed to see how they were radically destabilizing traditional relations between adults and children and thus eroding school discipline.

Attempts to Avoid Arbitrary, Capricious Decisions

School bureaucracies have struggled to restore the discipline that the courts and federal laws have taken away, but their efforts have only alienated students and undermined adult authority even more. Their first stratagem has been to bring in the lawyers to help them craft regulations, policies, and procedures. "If you have a law, you'd better have a policy," warns Julie Lewis, staff attorney for the American School Boards Association. These legalistic rules, designed more to avoid future lawsuits than to establish classroom order, are inevitably abstract and inflexible. Understandably, they inspire a certain contempt from students.

Putting them into practice often gives rise to the arbitrary and capricious decisions that lawmakers originally wanted to thwart. Take "zero tolerance" policies mandating automatic suspension of students for the worst offenses. These proliferated in the wake of Congress's 1994 Gun-Free Schools Act, which required school districts to boot out for a full year students caught with firearms. Many state and local boards, fearful that the federal law and the growing public clamor for safe schools could spawn a new generation of future lawsuits, fell into a kind of bureaucratic mania. Why not require suspension for *any* weapon—a nail file, a plastic Nerf gun? Common sense went out the window, and suspensions multiplied.

> *Students correctly sense that what lies behind [the] desiccated language [of school policies] is not a moral worldview and a concern for their well-being . . . but fear of lawsuits.*

Other districts wrote up new anti-weapon codes as precise and defensive as any corporate merger agreement. These efforts, however, ended up making educators look more obtuse. When a New York City high school student came to school with a metal-spiked ball whose sole purpose could only be to maim classmates, he wasn't suspended: metal-spiked balls weren't on the superintendent's detailed list of proscribed weapons. Suspend him, and he might sue you for being arbitrary and capricious.

Worse, the influence of lawyers over school discipline means that educators speak to children in an unrecognizable language, far removed from the straight talk about right and wrong that most children crave. A sample policy listed in "Keep Schools Safe," a pamphlet co-published by the National Attorneys General and the National School Boards Association (a partnership that itself says much about the character of American school discipline today), offers characteristically legalistic language: "I acknowledge and understand that 1. Student lockers are the property of the school system. 2. Student lockers remain at all times under the control of the school system. 3. I am expected to assume full responsibility for my school locker." Students correctly sense that what lies behind such desiccated language is not a moral worldview and a concern for their well-being and character but fear of lawsuits. . . .

Creating a Moral School Community

Good principals have to be a constant, palpable presence, out in the hallways, in the classrooms, in the cafeteria, enforcing and modeling for students and staff the moral ethos of the school. They're there, long before the school day begins and long after it ends; they know students' names, joke with them, and encourage them; and they don't let little things go—a nasty put-down between students, a profanity uttered in irritation, even a belt missing from a school uniform. They know which infraction takes only a gentle reminder and which a more forceful response—because they have a clear scale of values and they know their students. They work with their entire staff, from teachers to bus drivers, to enlist them in their efforts.

> *After Columbine, [numerous students] said they wouldn't bother reporting kids who had made threats or carried weapons because they didn't think [administrators] would do anything about them.*

For such principals, safety is of course a key concern. Frank Mickens, a wonderful principal of a big high school in a tough Brooklyn neighborhood, posts 17 staff members in the blocks near the school during dismissal time, while he sits in his car by the subway station, in order to keep students from fighting and bullies from picking on smaller or less aggressive children. Such measures go beyond reducing injuries. When students believe that the adults around them are not only fair but genuinely concerned with protecting them, the school can become a community that, like a good family, inspires affection, trust—and the longing to please.

But how can you create such a school if you have to make students sit next to felons or a kid transferred to your school because he likes to carry a box cutter in his pocket? June Arnette, Associate Director of the National School Safety Center, reports that, after Columbine, her office received numerous e-mails from students who said they wouldn't bother reporting kids who had made threats or carried weapons because they didn't think teachers or principals would do anything about them. A number of studies show that school officials rarely do anything about bullies.

How can you convince kids that you are interested in their well-being when from day one of the school year you feel bureaucratic pressure to speak to them in legalistic or quasi-therapeutic gobbledygook rather than a simple, moral language that they can understand? How can you inspire students' trust when you're not sure whether you can prevent a kid from wearing a WHITE POWER T-shirt or stop him from cursing at the teacher? It becomes virtually impossible, requiring heroic effort.

8

Students Are the Victims of Unjust School Policies

Advancement Project and Civil Rights Project

The Advancement Project collaborates with communities to build a fair, multiracial democracy in America and to advance opportunity, equity, and access for all. Founded in 1996 at Harvard University, the Civil Rights Project works to renew the civil rights movement by building a network of legal and social science scholars across the nation.

Although it is necessary to implement rules in order to protect students from harm, school policies have become increasingly callous and unfair. Zero tolerance policies, which require the suspension or expulsion of youths who possess weapons or drugs in school, have been expanded to include severe retribution for those who carry nail clippers, aspirin, and even breath mints, or who act childishly in class. Suspensions or expulsions for innocuous behavior are unnecessary disruptions in a child's education and may negatively affect his or her future opportunities. Worse, school policies are used to discriminate against African American, Latino, and Native American students, who are reprimanded by administrators more often than are whites. In addition, even though special-needs students cannot be legally punished for behavior caused by their disability, some have experienced rights violations by being expelled under harsh school policies and charged with felonies.

S chool safety is a critically important issue. Recent tragedies have heightened the public's fear and led to legitimate calls for stronger preventive measures. However, we must remember that "schools remain one of the safest places for children and youth," [according to the U.S. Safe and Drug-Free Schools Program.] Yet, the evidence gathered in this Report makes clear that efforts to address guns, drugs, and other truly dangerous school situations have spun totally out of control, sweeping up millions of schoolchildren who pose no threat to safety into a net of exclusion from educational opportunities and into criminal prosecution.

In a move to reduce the incidents of violence in public schools, several state legislatures, and subsequently Congress, passed laws implementing school disciplinary sanctions that became known as "Zero Tolerance Policies." These laws originally focused on truly dangerous and criminal behavior by students, requiring mandatory expulsion for possession of guns on school property. Many states later extended these laws to include other weapons and possession or use of drugs. School districts throughout the country quickly expanded Zero Tolerance Policies to include many more types of behavior and, significantly, to cover infractions that pose little or no safety concerns. Some of these policies employ sweeping interpretations of the federal law by including violations not intended to be covered by the laws. Aspirin, Midol, and even Certs have been treated as drugs, and paper clips, nail files, and scissors have been considered weapons. Other policies apply the theory of "Zero Tolerance" to a broad range of student actions that have absolutely no connection to violence and drugs. For example, last year [1999] Maryland schools (not including Baltimore City, the largest district) suspended 44,000 students for the non-violent offenses of "disobeying rules," "insubordination," and "disruption."

Students Are the Victims

In the strictest sense, these policies provide nondiscretionary punishment guidelines. However, they have become much more. Zero Tolerance has become a philosophy that has permeated our schools; it employs a brutally strict disciplinary model that embraces harsh punishment over education. As a result of this approach to discipline, students are losing out on educational opportunities. Case studies of middle schools in

Miami-Dade County [Florida] . . . demonstrate that where the zero tolerance philosophy is invoked, regardless of incidences of crime and violence, suspension rates are higher. [This] Report also indicates that even where schools experience repeated violations of codes of conduct, they can successfully employ solutions other than suspensions and expulsions. Of greater concern, this Report indicates that children are not only being treated like criminals in school, but many are being shunted into the criminal justice system as schools have begun to rely heavily upon law enforcement officials to punish students.

> *[Zero Tolerance] employs a brutally strict disciplinary model that embraces harsh punishment over education. As a result . . . , students are losing out on educational opportunities.*

School districts throughout the country are experiencing intense pressure to "keep learning in and trouble out." This pressure explains the comments made recently by Thomas Payzant, Superintendent of Boston Public Schools, justifying the suspension of a student for writing a horror story assigned by the teacher. "While school officials may not have the right answer, they have to err on the side of caution. . . . Maybe in the context of three or four years ago there wouldn't have been concern that embedded in this piece is perhaps a threat." Pedro Noguera, Professor of Education at the University of California, Berkeley, writes that these measures are "premised on the notion that violence in school can be reduced and controlled by identifying, apprehending and excluding violent or potentially violent individuals."

There Are More Effective Policies than Zero Tolerance

Yet, even in these fearful times, reasonable steps to protect students from guns, violence, and illegal drugs in their schools can be taken without resulting in the mass exclusion of American children from the educational process, which Zero Tolerance Policies are exacting. [Some] schools . . . are pursuing an alternative route to school safety. Recognizing that the vast majority of suspensions involve behaviors related to the interpersonal dynamics within the school, these schools are focusing on creating climates that facilitate "greater connections between adults and students," [Noguera reports.] Rather than concentrate on weeding out students who pose problems, they believe that most behaviors that might warrant exclusion from school can be prevented if students perceive themselves as valued and respected members of a larger community that nurtures strong relationships between school adults and students, sets high behavioral and academic standards, and values fairness and consistency. In other words, their efforts are geared toward eliminating certain behaviors, rather than the students themselves. Parents, students, activists, and policymakers should encourage school systems to adopt these positive and effective strategies.

The "Take No Prisoners" Approach

A zero tolerance story from the state of Mississippi exemplifies the extremely harsh disciplinary approach used in many school systems and the increasing invocation of the criminal justice system for minor school behavioral issues. At the beginning of [the 1999–2000] school year, students on a school bus were playfully throwing peanuts at one another. A peanut accidentally hit the white female bus driver, who immediately pulled over to call the police. After the police arrived, the bus was diverted to the courthouse, where children were questioned. Five African-American males, ages 17 and 18, were then arrested for felony assault, which carries a maximum penalty of five years in prison. The Sheriff commented to one newspaper, "[T]his time it was peanuts, but if we don't get a handle on it, the next time it could be bodies." The young men lost their bus privileges and suspension was recommended. As a result of the assistance of an attorney and community pressure, the criminal charges were dismissed. However, all five young men, who were juniors and seniors, dropped out of school because they lacked transportation to travel the 30 miles to their school in this poor, rural county in the Mississippi Delta. The impact of the punishment was underscored by one of the young men who stated, "I [would have] gone to college. . . . Maybe I could have been a lawyer." This story may be incredulous, but it is true; it epitomizes the recent overreaction to non-violent childish behavior, and the impact of senseless punishment.

Districts throughout the country have adopted a "take no prisoners" attitude toward discipline. As a result, more than 3.1 million students were suspended during the 1998 school year; another 87,000 were expelled. Although record-keeping and data availability on suspensions and expulsions is inadequate and inconsistent, the numbers that are available paint an extremely troubling picture. Last year [1999], in Jefferson County, Florida, a small, predominantly black school district, 43% of the high school students and 31% of middle school students were suspended at least once. In Wisconsin, suspensions have increased 34% since 1991–92; 25.5% of African-American males and 19.75% of Native American males were suspended during the 1997–98 school year. Chicago Public Schools have experienced a dramatic increase in the number of expulsions— an increase from 14 in 1992–93 to 737 in 1998–99. African-American students represent 73% of those expelled but only 53% of student enrollment; Latino students represent 20% of students expelled. Despite this disturbing situation in Chicago, the school district set a goal of expelling even more students during the 1999–2000 school year, bringing the number up to 1,500 students. In Florida, 3,831 students were referred to the Juvenile Justice system for conduct in school. The exclusion of students from the educational process is a crisis of epidemic proportions; it has long-term implications not only for the students affected, but also for our society as a whole.

Case Studies of Child "Criminals"

Statistics on the high number of students discarded from educational institutions do not fully tell the story of Zero Tolerance. These arbitrary, harsh rules are zealously applied to expel and suspend students—some as young as four years old—for trivial misconduct and innocent mistakes. While some of the most absurd of these stories have received media attention, thousands of others have not been exposed. The following is a sampling of reports from attorneys, advocates, and parents around the country that demonstrate the senselessness of zero tolerance and how these policies criminalize children.

• A six-year-old African-American child was suspended for ten days for bringing a toenail clipper to school. A school board member said, "This is not about a toenail clipper! This is about the attachments on the toenail clipper!" (Harrisburg, PA)

• A kindergarten boy in Pennsylvania was suspended for bringing a toy ax to school as part of his Halloween costume.

• A 14-year-old boy mistakenly left a pocketknife in his book bag after a Boy Scout camping trip. At his hearing, the boy's Scout Master testified on the boy's behalf. The student was expelled under the district's Zero Tolerance Policy, which requires expulsion for possession of knives. As a result of an appeal by Legal Aid Society of Greater Cincinnati, the student was readmitted to school, but had already missed 80 days of school. (OH)

> **"**[Problematic] behaviors . . . can be prevented if students perceive themselves as valued and respected members of a larger community that nurtures strong relationships between school adults and students . . . and values fairness.**"**

• A 4th grade ten-year-old African-American girl was charged with defiance of authority for failing to participate in a class assignment. She was suspended for three days. Soon thereafter, she was charged with "defiance of authority" for humming and tapping on her desk. She was again suspended for three days. She was subsequently suspended for five days for "defiance of authority" for talking back to her teacher and for "drug-related activity," namely, wearing one pants leg up, although there was no indication of any drug involvement. She was recommended for alternative school. The alternative school could not accept her because the alternative education system provides instruction for grades 5–12 only. The School District promoted her, despite her failing grades, in order to get her out of the mainstream school. Requests for a due process hearing have been denied. (MS)

• An African-American 9th grader was expelled for one year from a predominantly white school district and sent to an alternative school because she had sparklers in her book bag. She had used them over the weekend and forgot they were in her bag. (East Baton Rouge Parish, LA)

• An African-American male 7th grader bet a schoolmate on the outcome of a school basketball game. The schoolmate, who lost the bet, accused the boy of threatening him for payment. The school district conducted no investigation and instead notified law enforcement officials. The 7th grader was charged with felony extortion and expelled. (San Francisco, CA). . . .

A Pattern of Racial Inequities

Attorneys representing students in the disciplinary cases who were interviewed for this Report state that in their experience, African-American and Latino children are more likely [than whites] to be referred for disciplinary action and to be disciplined. In addition, these students are more likely to be disciplined for minor misconduct and to receive punishments disproportionate to their conduct. Attorneys also report that African-American and Latino children tend to be suspended for the more discretionary offenses, such as "defiance of authority" and "disrespect of authority." These categories of conduct clearly provide more latitude for racial bias to play a part in the use of disciplinary measures. Attorneys and community groups assert that school personnel rely upon racial and ethnic stereotypes in taking disciplinary actions. One attorney reported that she has often heard teachers comment about the size of black children accused of assault or battery.

> *These arbitrary, harsh rules are zealously applied to expel and suspend students—some as young as four years old—for trivial misconduct and innocent mistakes.*

The continuing pattern of racial disparities in school discipline is an issue that cannot be ignored. Regardless of whether intentional discrimination is the cause of the disproportionate suspension and expulsion of black and Latino children, the statistics are quite troubling. More research is needed to determine the cause of the disparities. In addition, the Department of Education's Office for Civil Rights, which is entrusted with enforcement of Title VI [which guarantees nondiscrimination in federally assisted programs], and the United States Commission on Civil Rights should vigorously investigate these disparities. It is imperative that innovative solutions to this problem be implemented. Our society cannot afford to leave any one segment of our population behind.

Children with Special
Needs Have Special Rights

Zero Tolerance Policies are also having a profound impact on children with special needs. In 1997, the Individuals with Disabilities Education Act (IDEA) was amended to ensure that a child would not be punished for behavior that was a characteristic of the child's disability. Although federal law provides this protection for special education students, school officials often unfairly discipline children with disabilities. For example:

• An autistic child hit a teacher. The child was expelled and charged with battery, which is a third degree felony. (Escambia County, FL)

• A ten-year-old child with a severe case of Attention Deficit Disorder was talking on the school bus and was told by the bus aide to be quiet or a written report would be filed. The child kicked the aide; he was arrested and charged with battery. (FL)

The amended IDEA provides extensive procedural protections for children with disabilities to ensure that under appropriate circumstances the impact of their disabilities are considered in meting out punishment, but in many circumstances, school officials are clearly ignoring the law. Furthermore, parents and students often are unaware of their rights or unable to enforce them.

9

Minors Should Have the Right to Vote

National Youth Rights Association

The National Youth Rights Association is a nonprofit group that defends the civil and human rights of American youths through education, empowerment, and cooperation with public officials.

In the United States the right to vote is denied to 16- and 17-year-olds even though they fulfill the same responsibilities as adults and thus should share the same rights. Because American teenagers pay taxes, follow laws, and are charged as adults when they commit serious crimes, they should have a voice in determining the the leaders who make the policies they must live under. Lowering the voting age to 16 would have numerous benefits; it would increase voter turnout, ensure that the needs of youths are served, prepare youths for a lifetime of voting, and strengthen democracy for all. Moreover, claims that teens would vote for the "wrong" candidates or elect dangerous radicals are unfounded. On the contrary, they, like most adult voters, would educate themselves on the issues before heading to the polls. Consequently, politicians should work toward granting the right to vote to 16- and 17-year-olds.

> "No right is more precious in a free country than that of having a choice in the election of those who make the laws under which . . . we must live. Other rights, even the most basic, are illusory if the right to vote is undermined."
>
> [—*Wesberry v. Saunders* (1964)]

In 1971 the United States ratified the 26th Amendment to the Constitution granting the right to vote to 18–20-year-olds. The 26th Amendment was the fastest to be ratified in U.S. history. At the height of the Vietnam War most Americans realized the sick double standard inherent in sending 18-year-old soldiers to fight and die for their country when they weren't allowed to vote. Double standards didn't go away in 1971. Right now youth are subject to adult penalties and even the death sentence[1] despite lacking the right to vote.

[Law professor] Frank Zimring found that "Between 1992 and 1995, forty American states relaxed the requirements for transferring an accused under the maximum age of jurisdiction into criminal court," and "In Colorado, for example, defendants under the maximum age for juvenile court jurisdiction may nonetheless be charged by direct filing in criminal court if they are over 14 years of age and are charged with one of a legislative list of violent crimes."

> *We tell youth they are judged mature, responsible adults when they commit murder, but silly, brainless kids when they want to vote?*

What kind of twisted message do we send when we tell youth they are judged mature, responsible adults when they commit murder, but silly, brainless kids when they want to vote? This is a double standard, no different than during the Vietnam War. War isn't a dead issue now either; leaders who youth can't vote for today may send them to war tomorrow. Lowering the voting age is the just, fair way to set things straight.

Because Youth Live Under Our Laws, They Should Have the Vote

Just like all other Americans, young Americans pay taxes. In fact, they pay a lot of taxes. Teens pay an estimated $9.7 billion dollars in sales taxes alone. Not to mention many millions of taxes on income. According to the IRS [Internal Revenue Service], "You may be a teen, you may not even have a permanent

1. In March 2005 capital punishment for juveniles was ruled unconstitutional.

job, but you have to pay taxes on the money you earn." Youth pay billions in taxes to state, local, and federal governments yet they have absolutely no say over how much is taken. This is what the American Revolution was fought over; this is taxation without representation.

In addition to being affected by taxes, young people are affected by every other law that Americans live under. As fellow citizens in this society, every action or inaction taken by lawmakers affects youth directly, yet they have no say in the matter. In her 1991 testimony before a Minnesota House subcommittee, 14-year-old Rebecca Tilsen had this to say:

> *Like all tax-paying, law-abiding Americans, youth must be given the right to vote.*

"If 16-year-olds are old enough to drink the water polluted by the industries that you regulate, if 16-year-olds are old enough to breathe the air ruined by garbage burners that government built, if 16-year-olds are old enough to walk on the streets made unsafe by terrible drugs and crime policies, if 16-year-olds are old enough to live in poverty in the richest country in the world, if 16-year-olds are old enough to get sick in a country with the worst public health-care programs in the world, and if 16-year-olds are old enough to attend school districts that you underfund, then 16-year-olds are old enough to play a part in making them better."

The just power of government comes from the consent of the governed: as it stands now youth are governed (overly so, some may say) but do not consent. This is un-American. Like all tax-paying, law-abiding Americans, youth must be given the right to vote. . . .

Lowering the Voting Age Will Increase Voter Turnout

For several reasons lowering the voting age will increase voter turnout. It is common knowledge that the earlier in life a habit is formed the more likely that habit or interest will continue throughout life. If attempts are made to prevent young people from picking up bad habits, why are no attempts made to get youth started with good habits, like voting? If citizens begin voting earlier, and get into the habit of doing so earlier, they are more likely to stick with it through life.

> *We do not deprive a senile person of this right [to vote], nor do we deprive any of the millions of alcoholics, neurotics, psychotics and assorted fanatics . . . of it.*

Not only will turnout increase for the remainder of young voters' lives, the turnout of their parents will increase as well. [We previously reported:] "A 1996 survey by Bruce Merrill, an Arizona State University journalism professor, found a strong increase in turnout. Merrill compared turnout of registered voters in five cities with Kids Voting with turnout in five cities without the program. Merrill found that between five and ten percent of respondents reported Kids Voting was a factor in their decision to vote. This indicated that 600,000 adults nationwide were encouraged to vote by the program."

Kids Voting is a program in which children participate in a mock vote and accompany their parents to the polls on Election Day. Reports show that even this modest gesture to [include] youth increased the [whole family's] interest in voting. . . . Parents were more likely to discuss politics with their kids and thus an estimated 600,000 adult voters were more likely to vote because of it. Lowering the voting age will strengthen this democracy for all of us.

If We Let Stupid Adults Vote, Why Not Let Smart Youth Vote?

[According to consultant Richard Farson,] the argument that youth "should not vote because they lack the ability to make informed and intelligent decisions is valid only if that standard is applied to all citizens." But yet this standard is not applied to all citizens, only young people. [Farson points out,] "We do not deprive a senile person of this right, nor do we deprive any of the millions of alcoholics, neurotics, psychotics and assorted fanatics who live outside hospitals of it. We seldom ever prevent those who are hospitalized for mental illness from voting."

Even beyond senile, neurotic, and psychotic adults, regular adults often do not meet the unrealistic standard opponents to youth voting propose. Turn on the *Tonight Show* one night and see the collection of adult buffoons who can't tell [host] Jay Leno who the vice-president is, or who have forgotten how many states are in this country. Yet these adults are happily given the right to vote. The fact is, intelligence or maturity is not the basis upon which the right to vote is granted; if that were the case all voters would need to pass a test before voting. [However,] ". . . under voting rights jurisprudence, literacy tests are highly suspect (and indeed are banned under federal law), and lack of education or information about election issues is not a basis for withholding the franchise," [according to *Children in the Legal System: Cases and Materials*.] Youth shouldn't be held to a stricter standard than adults; lower the voting age.

Youth Will Vote Well

It is silly to fear that huge masses of youth will rush to the voting booth and unwittingly vote for Mickey Mouse and Britney Spears. By and large, those individuals with no interest in politics and no knowledge on the subject will stay home from the polls and not vote. This mechanism works for adult voters as well. Youth will behave no differently.

> *It is silly to fear that huge masses of youth will rush to the voting booth and unwittingly vote for Mickey Mouse and Britney Spears.*

Besides foolishly throwing a vote away, some worry about youth voting for dangerous radicals. These fears are unfounded as well. [As child education specialist John Holt writes,] "We should remember, too, that many people today vote at first, and often for many years after, exactly as their parents voted. We are all deeply influenced, in politics as everything else, by the words and example of people we love and trust." One's political leanings are influenced by their community and their family, and it is likely young voters will vote in much the same way as their parents, not because they are coerced to do so, but because of shared values.

With the voting age at 16 . . . new voters [will] have a greater opportunity to be educated [about voting] in high school. When the voting age is lowered schools will most likely schedule a civics class to coincide with 16 that will introduce the issues and prepare new voters. It stands to reason that these young voters will be better prepared to vote than their elders.

There Are No Wrong Votes

Noting that youth will most likely vote well we must wonder, is it at all possible for a voter to vote wrong? Did voters choose poorly when they elected [President Bill] Clinton in 1992? Republicans would say so. Did voters choose poorly when they elected [President George W.] Bush in 2000? Democrats would say so. If youth were able to vote for either of them, or against them, would they be voting wrong? I don't think so. All voters have their own reasons for voting. We may disagree with their reasons, but we must respect their right to make a decision. This is what we must do with youth.

Lowering the Voting Age Will Provide an Intrinsic Benefit to Youth

Granting youth the right to vote will have a direct effect on their character, intelligence and sense of responsibility. Is it any wonder why many youth feel apathetic towards politics? After 18 years of . . . being told their opinion doesn't matter, they are just foolish children who should be seen and not heard, is anyone surprised that many people over 18 feel turned off by politics and don't vote? We can see this contrast between volunteering and politics. Teenagers have amazingly high levels of volunteering and community service, however many feel turned off by politics. Even small gestures like mock voting has a large effect on teen's interest in politics. [In our "Proposal to Lower the Voting Age," we noted that] of students participating in Kids Voting USA, "More than 71% of students reported frequently or occasionally questioning parents about elections at home. These same students also viewed voting with great importance. About 94% felt it was very important or somewhat important to vote." Including youth in a real, substantive way in politics will lead to even more interest as they take their public-spirited nature into the political realm.

Many opponents to lowering the voting age assume apathetic youth today will be no different when given the right to vote: this is wrong. Responsibility comes with rights, not the other way around. [Philospher Avrum Stroll contends,] "It is not a pre-condition of self-government that those that govern be wise, educated, mature, responsible and so on, but instead these are the results which self-government is designed to produce." Educator and youth rights theorist John Holt points out that if youth "think their choices and decisions make a difference to them, in their own lives, they will have every reason to try to choose and decide more wisely. But if what they think makes no difference, why bother to think?" He stresses this point again, "It is not just power, but impotence, that corrupts people. It gives them the mind and soul of slaves. It makes them indifferent, lazy, cynical, irresponsible, and, above all, stupid."

Lowering the voting age may not be the magic bullet to improve the lives of youth, but by giving them a real stake in their futures and their present lives it will push them to become involved, active citizens of this great nation. The National Youth Rights Association strongly urges lawmakers and individuals in this country to seriously consider lowering the voting age.

10

Minors Should Not Be Permitted to Vote

Ellie Levenson

Ellie Levenson is a freelance journalist and former editor of Fabian Review, *a publication of the Fabian Society, a left-leaning United Kingdom think tank.*

In 2004 the United Kingdom considered lowering its voting age from 18 to 16. This was a gaffe because the majority of teenagers would not vote even if they were permitted to and certainly do not have the maturity to make such important decisions. If given the vote, many teenagers would vote rebelliously rather than responsibly. While some people assert that 16-year-olds can consent to have sex, get married, and join the military and therefore should also have the right to vote, it should be noted that most minors are not responsible enough to do any of those things. Some youths, of course, would take voting seriously, but it is necessary to choose a minimum voting age at which nearly *everyone* is mature—such as 25 years of age.

To be against lowering the voting age is seen by most progressives as symptomatic of losing one's youth and gaining some grumpiness. So for a relatively young progressive such as myself to be against lowering the voting age—well, I might as well have said let's abolish the vote altogether going by the looks I have received from many of my colleagues on the left.

The Electoral Commission releases its report on lowering the voting age today [April 19, 2004], and if [Great Britain's] Labour Party's growing sympathy towards this idea is anything

82

to go by, it is likely that it will come out in favour of it.[1]

This is a mistake, for two reasons. The first is that it is a simple case of ostrich head meets sand. Yes it is a sad fact that over 40 per cent of those eligible to vote in this country [Great Britain] did not exercise their right to do so in the last general election. It's generally agreed that this constitutes some kind of crisis of political engagement. However, by increasing the number of people eligible to vote you merely have the same percentage of a larger number of people not voting, or perhaps an even larger percentage of people not voting, as the youngest group of eligible voters usually has the lowest turnout.

Sixteen-Year-Olds Are Too Immature to Vote

But the second reason, and most important one, is that the majority of 16-year-olds are just not responsible enough or mature enough to have the vote.

Those who argue against this use the bundling of rights argument: the age of consent is 16, people can get married at 16, people can join the armed forces at 16, and that there should be no taxation without representation. Therefore, they think, it follows that 16-year-olds should also have the vote.

Well, we know that just because a person has sex does not mean that they are responsible. Look at Britain's teen pregnancy rate. There seems little logical connection between having the right to participate in sex and having the right to vote. Animals, after all, have sex, yet we do not propose giving our pets the vote.

> *There seems little logical connection between having the right to participate in sex and having the right to vote. Animals . . . have sex, yet we do not propose giving our pets the vote.*

To get married in England and Wales people under 18 require parental consent. Do we want people to ask for parental consent to vote for a party of their choice? And how many of us really think a 16-year-old is capable of making a life-changing

1. It recommended leaving the voting age at 18.

and legally binding decision such as marriage? Financial institutions certainly do not think so. You must be 18 to sign binding contracts or to own land in your own name. Therefore 16-year-olds, married with parental permission or not, cannot apply for a mortgage or own the house in which they live.

> *Perhaps 'should we lower the voting age?' is the wrong question. Instead it should be should we raise it?*

Similarly, under 18s need parental consent to join the armed forces, and in normal circumstances are not deployed on operations until they are 18. In fact, the UN [United Nations] supports raising the age of joining the forces to 18.

As for no taxation without representation, all young people pay tax if they spend money—VAT [value-added tax]. A 10-year-old spending their pocket money on a burger in McDonald's or on a CD pays tax. Does this mean they should be given the vote? Or does this argument just refer to income tax, in which case, if tax is so inextricably tied up with voting rights, do they think the vote should be taken away from those whose incomes do not reach the threshold for paying income tax?

Teens Are Too Rebellious

But whether or not a taxpayer, spouse, parent or soldier, 16-year-olds should not have the vote.

It is during a person's teenage years that they are most likely to be exposed to new ideas and points of view, be it through school, the new people they meet or from the media. This is the age at which people should be able to think through their political ideas and change them at will, debate and try out policies without having to act on them and without having to take responsibility for their ideas.

And it is at this age that teenagers are at their most rebellious and negative stage, a time when they are more keen on making a statement than acting responsibly. Rebellion against your parents' taste in music and their rules is one thing; let's not make that part of the democratic process by which our government is elected.

As we all know, maturity rates in teenagers differ tremendously, both in terms of the ability to think through an argument logically and in terms of the ability to understand cause and effect and to take responsibility for their own actions. Some 16-years-olds look and act as if they are in their twenties. Others are still childlike and unable to take on responsibility or act independently.

Voting is a serious matter. It is what makes a democracy, and must be taken seriously by all voters. I don't think most 16-year-olds are mature enough to vote. Some will be capable of voting (and having sex, getting married and joining the armed forces) at 16—others will not be ready at 18. As the law must be arbitrary, we need the highest common denominator, and 18 is a better line than 16.

So perhaps "should we lower the voting age?" is the wrong question. Instead it should be should we raise it, and if so, to what age? I am 25. I think this would be a good age.

11

Children Do Not Have the Right to Join an Army

Sarah Rose Miller

This essay by teenager Sarah Rose Miller earned honorable mention in the 2001 Humanist *Essay Contest for Young Women and Men of North America.*

Armies have conscripted hundreds of thousands of children as young as seven years old to serve as soldiers or as prostitutes for soldiers. Whether youths join a militia voluntarily or are forcibly recruited, their service is an unconscionable abuse of human rights. Because minors are too young to understand how stressful and horrific war is, they should never be permitted to join the armed forces; youths who wish to support a cause should choose nonviolent means instead. Yet more than three hundred thousand children remain involved in armed conflicts throughout the world, and millions more have been killed, disfigured, or emotionally scarred from combat. Those who survive and are released from service frequently have trouble assimilating into society. Traumatized and unable to interact with others, many former child soldiers become involved in prostitution. In response to the child soldiery epidemic, the U.S. government must support efforts to reintegrate all child soldiers into civilian life.

There are armed conflicts going on all over the world, and not only adults but children are suffering and dying. And

Sarah Rose Miller, "Child Soldiers," *Humanist*, vol. 62, July/August 2002. Copyright © 2002 by the *Humanist*. Reproduced by permission.

it's not only those children who happen to be in the wrong place at the wrong time when enemy soldiers come through or when a bomb is dropped on civilian establishments. Children are marching, fighting, killing, and dying—seventeen year olds, thirteen year olds, and youths as young as seven, who may not even understand what they are fighting for. It's sad that today, in the twenty-first century, children are still being used in such a way. It is disgraceful that people all over the world stand by and watch as children die for them. This can and must end.

Why Children Join Armies

According to the U.S. Campaign to Stop the Use of Child Soldiers, the number of children under the age of eighteen who are at this time [in 2002] involved in armed conflicts throughout the world is over 300,000, and hundreds of thousands more could be sent to fight at any moment. An estimated two million youths have been killed in combat in the past decade [1992–2002] alone, and three times as many have been seriously wounded or disfigured.

Some children join the army voluntarily, many of them from poverty-stricken homes with lives of hardship. For some, the army may provide a better life than they are accustomed to. They can get regular meals and wages or escape from an abusive home environment. But children in the army are frequently abused and harassed there, and the promise of minimal food and money often isn't worth the cost: lifelong trauma, physical disabilities, or death.

> *The [army's] promise of minimal food and money often isn't worth the cost: lifelong trauma, physical disabilities, or death.*

Children also join armed forces for other reasons, the most common being that it is practically a custom within their culture. They may feel passionately about a particular cause and see this as an opportunity to support it, or they may be insecure and feel the need to have control of a weapon. Being in the military may help raise a youth's confidence, if not mistreated or called into battle. Sometimes it isn't the child's choice at all. Occasionally parents volunteer their children for recruitment into the armed forces, and youths have also been abducted, press-ganged, or otherwise forcibly conscripted into the military.

Children's Usefulness in War

Child soldiers are actually preferred by some army commanders because they are easier to manage and manipulate than adults. They aren't as likely to question orders. So, in the case of children, the commanding officer is clearly the power behind the guns, whereas adult soldiers are more likely to disobey orders, thereby detracting from the authority of the commander. Children are also more likely to carry out suicide missions than are adults.

> *Children are . . . more likely to carry out suicide missions than are adults.*

The downside to child soldiers on a military level is that they are generally weaker than adults, both physically and mentally. They are more likely to be unable to sustain long marches or strenuous missions or carry heavy loads (which, despite their unsuitability, is often what they are forced to do). Children aren't as desensitized to violence; being less callous, they may be unable to continue when exposed to the horrors of battle. Stressful assignments or situations undermine a child's fortitude, and abuse from fellow soldiers and commanders, which often occurs, can severely traumatize a child or teen.

Child soldiers—mainly girls but occasionally boys too—are often sexually exploited. Whether this is done to distract adult soldiers from the horrors of war, to merely have some fun, or both, this sort of treatment can haunt children their whole lives. One girl from Honduras, who had served in the army, later said:

> At the age of thirteen, I joined the student movement. I had a dream to contribute to make things change, so that children would not be hungry. . . .
> Later I joined the armed struggle. I had all the inex-

perience and the fears of a little girl. I found out that girls were obliged to have sexual relations "to alleviate the sadness of the combatants." And who alleviated our sadness after going with someone we hardly knew? At my young age I experienced abortion. It was not my decision. There is a great pain in my being when I recall all these things. . . . In spite of my commitment, they abused me; they trampled my human dignity. And above all they did not understand that I was a child and that I had rights.

Immoral and Unconscionable

Not all child soldiers are mistreated, harassed, or manipulated; some are protected and cared for. But no matter how much a child in the army is sheltered, all the pain and horror of war cannot be hidden. When a war is going on, commanders will send children into battle eventually. It is inevitable that they will witness—or worse, experience—atrocities that most other children can only have nightmares about.

Some people might maintain that the end is worth the means. If the cause that children are fighting for is a good one, perhaps it will save lives in the long run. It is possible that having a few hundred more soldiers on one side in a certain battle could be the difference between winning and losing a war—but it is improbable. It is much more likely that hundreds of youths will die in a battle that makes no ultimate difference whatsoever. Furthermore, it can work both ways: children can also support an unjust cause. Whichever the case, allowing so many children to die is a means that can never be justified by such an extremely dubious end. For even the noblest end, the means of child soldiery is both immoral and unconscionable.

> *They trampled my human dignity. And above all they did not understand that I was a child and that I had rights.*

Do adults have the right to tell youths that they cannot stand up for their views—that they must let adults handle the conflict for them? There are other ways to support a view than to wield a weapon and kill those you oppose; fighting is not necessarily the best solution. In an ideal world, there would be no war, no violence. And although this isn't and never will be an ideal world, people can strive toward this vision by finding nonviolent ways to support their beliefs. Perhaps recognizing that the use of child soldiers can never be justified will be a first step toward the recognition that no one should be a soldier. Still, in a world in which wars are seen as legitimate, can adults rightly forbid children to join in them? Perhaps the most important reason for doing so is that children can have no real idea of what they are consenting to. When they join up, few children are aware of what being in an army actually entails. By the time reality sets in, desertion is the only means of escape.

> *Whether it is or isn't their choice [to join the army, children] don't deserve to be forfeiting their lives.*

Child soldiers who survive often have a difficult time assimilating to society. They may be physically disabled or emotionally scarred and, having spent years of their lives training and fighting, may be unused to interacting within a social community. Studies show that a large number of former child soldiers become victims of prostitution. Youths frequently return home to discover their families are no longer alive or have dissolved. And even if the family is still alive and together, children are often unable to bridge the gap caused by years of separation and different lifestyles.

One of the current situations involving the use of child soldiers is the West Asian crisis. Afghan military units have been using children as soldiers for twenty years, raising and educating them in extremely militaristic schools and environments and utilizing them in the civil wars. Large numbers of children were recruited by the Taliban from a particular type of religious school in Pakistan called a *madrasa*. Madrasas are mainly for poor students who can afford little better, and many Afghan refugees attend them. The al-Qaeda [terrorists] were long rumored to have been recruiting children and training them for military combat; therefore many of the youths injured and killed during U.S. military activities against al-

Qaeda and Taliban forces were likely in the service of [al-Qaeda founder] Osama bin Laden's troops.

Child Soldiering Endangers the Future of Humanity

There are a number of national and international efforts to stop the use of child soldiers. The U.S. Campaign to Stop the Use of Child Soldiers upholds an international ban on recruitment of youths under eighteen years of age for armed services. Its aims are:

• U.S. ratification of the new child soldiers protocol [developed by the United Nations]

• elimination of U.S. military aid that facilitates the use of child soldiers by other governments or armed political groups

• increased U.S. governmental and nongovernmental support for programs to prevent child recruitment and to provide for the demobilization, rehabilitation, and social reintegration of child soldiers

• raising the U.S. enlistment age to eighteen.

Anti–child soldier organizations in other countries have similar goals, adjusted to the circumstances of their own nations.

We, the people of the world, adults and children alike—those who are soldiers as well as those who aren't—must support these organizations. We must acknowledge that children the world over are fighting, bleeding, suffering, and dying for us. Whether it is or isn't their choice, they don't deserve to be forfeiting their lives which have only just been embarked upon. Many children who aren't soldiers have to face death too—due to accidents, disease, or some other natural cause. But soldiering isn't natural. It's the result of people standing by while youths risk everything. These children are the future of humanity and, by endangering them, we endanger our own future.

12

Circumcision of Young Girls Violates Their Rights

NotJustSkin

As an educational nonprofit organization, NotJustSkin provides information about questionable medical procedures and advocates human rights.

Female circumcision, or female genital cutting (FGC), is a procedure performed on girls mainly from Africa and the Middle East for religious and cultural reasons. It has been identified by the United Nations and other world organizations as a human rights abuse. The procedure involves the partial or total amputation of a female child's clitoris, labia majora, and labia minora. In its most extreme form, FGC also includes the almost total closing of the vulva, leaving a vaginal opening so small that women must later undergo surgery in order to deliver a child. Sometimes performed using unsterilized instruments such as pieces of glass, female circumcision causes severe pain and psychological trauma. It carries a risk of infection, blood loss, shock, and death, as well as long-term complications, including loss of sexual sensation, pain during intercourse, and chronic infections. Furthermore, genital cutting violates a child's right to bodily integrity and to informed consent. People should be educated about the procedure's harms in order to eradicate this highly damaging practice.

In many cultural traditions, body modification rituals are performed on children. Among the most common of these rituals are those involving cutting the genitals of children. These rituals, female genital cutting (FGC) and male genital cutting (MGC), damage the sexual organs and have many complications.

FGC, also called female circumcision, is practiced by diverse peoples, including Muslims and Christians, on girls ranging in age from infancy to the late teenage years. Specifics of the practice vary more by tribal/cultural affiliation than by national border. FGC is usually a ritual of great cultural significance performed by an older woman in the community.

An estimated 130 million women and girls alive today have been subjected to FGC. Eight to ten million girls and women in the Middle East and Africa, and thousands in the U.S., are currently at risk for FGC.

Types and Risks of Female Genital Cutting

There are three main types of FGC. Type I, also called Sunna circumcision, is the amputation of the tip or hood of the clitoris. (This procedure is often represented as removal of the entire clitoris due to a misconception of clitoral anatomy.) This form of FGC is the most widely practiced, and accounts for about 80% of FGC incidents.

> *The instruments (such as razor blades, scissors, or pieces of glass) in many cases are not sterilized and may be used on several children in succession.*

Type II FGC is the amputation of part or all of the clitoris and scraping away of parts of the labia majora and labia minora. This form is practiced mostly in regions where infibulation is becoming illegal or discouraged.

Type III FGC, also called infibulation or pharaonic circumcision, is the complete amputation of the clitoris, labia majora, and labia minora, and sewing together of the sides of the vulva with thorns, catgut, or some other suturing material. A small opening is left for the passage of menstrual fluids and urine.

According to one estimate, in 1992 infibulation was universal throughout Somalia and in populations of ethnic Somalians in Ethiopia, Kenya and Djibouti; throughout the Nile Valley, including Southern Egypt; and along the Red Sea Coast.

> *[Historically, circumcision was] performed on boys and girls with the explicit purpose of causing pain to the genitals and diminishing sexual pleasure.*

Consequences of MGC and Type I FGC can include scarring, loss of blood, infection, shock, and death, and later, painful intercourse for both partners and reduced ability to experience sexual pleasure. MGC and FGC are also potential vectors of disease transmission, including HIV, since the instruments (such as razor blades, scissors, or pieces of glass) in many cases are not sterilized and may be used on several children in succession.

Additional long-term complications of Type II and III FGC can include delayed menarche, chronic pelvic problems, damaged birth canal, and recurrent urinary retention and infection. Women who have been infibulated may experience yet more severe complications and must undergo an operation to allow the passage of the child during labor.

One of the few doctors in the U.S. who has experience treating complications of FGC, Dr. Nahid Toubia, has written a guide to caring for women subjected to FGC.

Anecdotal accounts indicate that FGC can lead to long-term physical and psychological harm.

FGC Is Illegal in the United States and Other Countries

The U.S. Federal Prohibition of Female Genital Mutilation Act of 1995 illegalizes any surgical procedure on the sexual organs of a girl before age 18, regardless of cultural or religious beliefs, unless the procedure is deemed "medically necessary" and performed by a licensed physician. FGC is punishable by a fine or prison sentence [of] up to 5 years. Sixteen states have passed additional laws against circumcision of female minors. Some activists and lawyers note that these laws, which offer no protection to male minors, are sex-discriminatory.

FGC is still practiced in the U.S., primarily within certain recently immigrated groups. On January 9, 2004, the Associated Press reported the arrest of a California couple who allegedly have performed numerous female circumcisions. The case is the first to be filed under the federal 1995 law.

There are laws against FGC in Australia, Britain, Canada, France, Sweden, Switzerland, New Zealand, Burkina Faso, Cote d'Ivoire, Kenya, Sudan, and Senegal. Some of these laws forbid only certain forms of FGC and many are not enforced. Immigrants are known to practice FGC in Australia, Canada, New Zealand, the U.S. and in European nations. In Egypt, FGC is legal only when performed by medical professionals in a hospital setting. Hospital FGC may remove more tissue.

Female Genital Cutting in Context

Ritual alteration of children's bodies has been a common phenomenon throughout history, from footbinding to head flattening to various forms of scarification. However, genital cutting may be the only such ritual to have become incorporated into mainstream medical practice.

In the late 1800's, the practices of MGC and type I FGC rapidly gained popularity in the medical institutions of English speaking countries. Circumcision and other procedures were performed on boys and girls with the explicit purpose of causing pain to the genitals and diminishing sexual pleasure.

Physicians recognized that the foreskin of the penis and the clitoral tip of the vulva are dense concentrations of specialized, erogenous nerves. Sexual excitation was at the time considered a dangerous form of nervous excitement, responsible for many ailments. As one physician [Jonathan Hutchinson] wrote, voicing increasingly popular medical opinion in 1891, more radical procedures would "be a true kindness to many patients of both sexes."

FGC eventually lost popularity. However, mainstream medical journals published articles advocating adult FGC as late as 1959 [such as "Female Circumcision: Indications and a New Technique," *General Practitioner*, September 1959].

Male genital cutting, also called male circumcision, continues to be performed in the U.S., principally on infants.

Genital alteration surgeries also continue to be performed

on children with intersex conditions. Intersex is a catchall term for several conditions in which an individual is born with atypical reproductive or sexual anatomy. Children identified as intersex are not protected by the 1995 FGC law and may be subjected to clitoral reduction or other forced gender assignment surgeries in an attempt to normalize their appearance.

Internationally, MGC occurs almost everywhere FGC occurs, while the reverse is not true. Two percent of the world's women, and fifteen percent of the world's men have been subjected to genital cutting. Within a given culture, both procedures tend to take place under similar conditions, such as the use of unhygienic instruments, lack of anesthetic, and the discouragement or shaming of emotional expressions.

FGC and MGC typically serve parallel social functions, such as rites of adulthood, preparation for marriage, and responses to myths that the genitals are unclean and cause disease. Usually the rituals are administered by practitioners of the same gender as the child.

Both MGC and FGC remove healthy, sexually specialized tissue from children, have short-term risks such as infection, and have long-term sexual complications. People subjected to child genital cutting have publicly denounced the practices and asserted that they cause psychological harm.

> *Child genital cutting violates the individual's rights to physical and mental health, self-determination, [and] bodily integrity.*

Comparisons of MGC and FGC are difficult. Male circumcision removes an adult equivalent 12–15 square inches of epidermis, the subcutaneous dartos muscle, and 10,000–20,000 nerve endings. Type I FGC removes several thousand nerve endings but far less tissue. Typical Type II FGC removes much of the external tissue, 10,000–20,000 nerve endings, and may result in additional complications related to childbirth. Type III FGC, castration, and subincision (a type of MGC involving a cut from the head of the penis toward the base), can have severe reproductive consequences and the greatest risks for infection and hemorrhage. All of these procedures are performed with instruments ranging from aseptic scalpels to rusted blades.

[Researcher] Hanny Lightfoot-Klein pioneered the first in-depth study of the widespread practice of infibulation in Sub-Saharan Africa. During her six year study, she lived with families and interviewed over 400 people in all social levels about FGC. At the Third International Symposium on Circumcision, she compared the practice and its motivations to infant circumcision in the U.S.:

> . . . the more insight I gained into the various forms of genital mutilation of children, both in the pre-scientific societies I studied in Africa and the technologically advanced United States, the more I was struck by the similarities in rationale structures invented and proliferated by both . . . to trivialize and justify the damage they contrived to perpetrate upon the bodies and psyches of their non-consenting and defenseless offspring.

Child Genital Cutting as a Human Rights Issue

Child genital cutting violates the individual's rights to physical and mental health, self-determination, bodily integrity, and freedom from sex discrimination. However, only FGC is acknowledged as a serious human rights violation by the United Nations [U.N.], UNICEF [United Nations Children's Fund], the World Health Organization, and Amnesty International.

> *[In genital cutting] attention is diverted from children's rights to the parent's right to choose, to a collection of medical or hygienic myths, [or] to freedom of religion.*

U.N. resolutions establishing these rights include:
- Universal Declaration on Human Rights (1948)
- International Covenant on Civil & Political Rights (1966)
- Convention on the Rights of the Child (1989)

In addition, when performed as a medical procedure, genital cutting typically violates the right to informed consent because the sexual effects of the surgery are usually ignored, the potential complications minimized, and dubious benefits emphasized.

Within cultures practicing FGC or MGC, attention is diverted from children's rights to the parent's right to choose, to a collection of medical or hygienic myths, to freedom of religion, or the issue is taboo or simply ignored. Human rights are seen as inapplicable to the local genital cutting ritual.

Toward the End of Child Genital Cutting

Outlawing common practices such as FGC is problematic and has not proven successful. A more successful approach has been to introduce alternative rituals that address cultural needs but do not involve bloodletting and to offer practitioners, whose income may be largely from FGC, jobs as health educators in exchange for ceasing to perform FGC.

Challenges to ending FGC are presented by the cultural biases of the activists who target the issue. Outsiders can be perceived as insulting and confusing when they speak without understanding the relevant cultural framework, when they hold a viewpoint in which tribal beliefs are less significant than their own religions, or when they deal with FGC while ignoring MGC. Even parents who have immigrated to the U.S. may have trouble understanding prohibitions against FGC partly because mainstream religions and medical practices call for the circumcision of boys.

Describing FGC and MGC as "mutilation" is discouraged because it tends to polarize discussion and be seen as culturally bigoted. People who have been subjected to these procedures also may not prefer to identify [themselves] as "mutilated."

Grassroots education appears to be key to eliminating child genital cutting. There can be strong resistance to ending practices that have always been presented as positive, or at least benign. However, a personal, informative, non-threatening approach that encourages self-empowerment can be effective. Educators can raise awareness about the harmful aspects of genital cutting, debunk myths about genital cutting, provide accurate medical information, and encourage people to change social pressure by supporting human rights. Framing the discussion so that the benefits of ceasing the practice outweigh the costs *from the decision maker's point of view* is essential.

[Sociologist] Gerry Mackie asserts FGC has such a high level of social importance that "an individual in an intramarrying group that practices FGC can't give it up unless enough other people do too." Mackie suggests that the three steps to ending

FGC are to provide an alternative rite of passage, publicize the health benefits of naturalism and the risks of FGC, and form societies that pledge not to perform FGC.

An International Coalition for Genital Integrity has formed to provide a resource and common voice to organizations opposing non-consenting child genital surgeries.

13

Children Have a Right to Online Privacy

Federal Trade Commission

The Federal Trade Commission (FTC) is the U.S. govern-
ment agency that works to protect consumers from unfair or
deceptive marketplace practices.

In the past, youths were prompted to disclose their name,
address, age, and other identifiable information to Web
site operators without the knowledge or consent of their
parents. Today the Children's Online Privacy Protection
Act (COPPA) is successfully preserving children's right to
online privacy. Initiated in 1998, the legislation places restrictions on any Web site or online service that is aimed
at youths under thirteen or that knowingly collects personal information from minors. Under the law these sites
must obtain a parent's or guardian's permission before
collecting a child's data, cannot ask children to disclose
more personal information than is reasonably necessary,
and must inform parents or guardians of their right to review or delete information collected from their child.
Since its inception, COPPA has been used to prosecute six
cases of privacy rule violations, and the majority of Internet sites that gather children's personal information now
have established privacy policies. The government took
further steps in 2002 to ensure that Web site operators
knew how to become COPPA compliant, making certain
that children's privacy is protected.

O n the second anniversary of the Children's Online Privacy
Protection Rule [which became effective in April 2000],

Federal Trade Commission, "FTC Protecting Children's Privacy Online," www.ftc.
gov, April 22, 2002.

the Federal Trade Commission [FTC] announced its sixth COPPA [the Children's Online Privacy Protection Act of 1998] enforcement case together with new initiatives designed to enhance compliance with the law.

The package of initiatives includes:

• A settlement with the operators of the Etch-A-Sketch Web site resolving alleged violations of COPPA and requiring a $35,000 civil penalty;

• Release of an FTC COPPA compliance survey, and a business education initiative to help children's Web site operators draft COPPA-compliant privacy policies;

• Announcement of warning letters to more than 50 children's sites alerting them to the notice provisions of COPPA and the requirement that they comply with these provisions; and

• Extension of COPPA's sliding scale mechanism for obtaining verifiable parental consent for a three year period.

Preserving Children's Privacy

"Enforcing promises to protect the personal information of our youngest consumers is an important part of our privacy program," said J. Howard Beales, III, Director of the FTC's Bureau of Consumer Protection. "With the publication of the COPPA privacy policy compliance guide, Web sites that cater to kids have a new plain language guide to how to get it right."

> *Enforcing promises to protect the personal information of our youngest consumers is an important part of our privacy program.*

The Children's Online Privacy Protection Act applies to operators of commercial Web sites and online services directed to children under the age of 13, and to general audience Web sites and online services that knowingly collect personal information from children. Among other things, the law requires that Web sites obtain verifiable consent from a parent or guardian before they collect personal information from children. It also prohibits sites from conditioning a child's participation in an activity on the child's disclosing more personal information than is reasonably necessary to participate in such an activity.

The Ohio Art Company, manufacturer of the Etch-A-Sketch drawing toy, will pay $35,000 to settle Federal Trade Commission charges that it violated the Children's Online Privacy Protection Rule by collecting personal information from children on its www.etch-a-sketch.com Web site without first obtaining parental consent. The settlement also bars future violations of the COPPA Rule. This is the FTC's sixth COPPA law enforcement case.

> *The site collected the names, mailing addresses, e-mail addresses, age, and date of birth from children who wanted to qualify to win an Etch-A-Sketch.*

The FTC alleges that The Ohio Art Company collected personal information from children registering for "Etchy's Birthday Club." The site collected the names, mailing addresses, e-mail addresses, age, and date of birth from children who wanted to qualify to win an Etch-A-Sketch toy on their birthday. The FTC charged that the company merely directed children to "get your parent or guardian's permission first," and then collected the information without first obtaining parental consent as required by the law. In addition, the FTC alleged that the company collected more information from children than was reasonably necessary for children to participate in the "birthday club" activity, and that the site's privacy policy statement did not clearly or completely disclose all of its information collection practices or make certain disclosures required by COPPA. The site also failed to provide parents the opportunity to review the personal information collected from their children and to inform them of their ability to prevent the further collection and use of this information, the FTC alleged.

Efforts to Ensure Compliance with COPPA

The agency also announced the results of an April 2001 COPPA compliance survey reviewing information collection practices at 144 children's Web sites. The 2001 survey follows up on an earlier 1998 survey and indicates that much progress has been made. For example, the vast majority—nearly 90 percent—of the sites that collected personal information from children had privacy policies, as opposed to only 24 percent in 1998. At the same time, the survey shows that many sites are not fully complying with all the requirements of the Rule. For example, only about half the sites complied with COPPA-specific notice requirements such as informing parents of their right to review information collected from their child, have it deleted, and to refuse to allow further collection of information.

> **"** *[By 2001] nearly 90 percent . . . of the sites that collected personal information from children had privacy policies, as opposed to only 24 percent in 1998.* **"**

To improve compliance, the FTC has launched an educational effort and issued a new publication, *You, Your Privacy Policy and COPPA*, to assist the operators of children's Web sites in drafting a COPPA-compliant privacy policy. This guide explains each component of a COPPA-compliant privacy policy, answers questions that Web site operators have asked, and features a compliance checklist to help site operators improve their privacy policies.

The FTC also has sent letters to more than 50 children's Web site operators, identified through its April 2001 survey, warning them that they must improve their privacy policies in order to make them COPPA compliant. The site operators were sent copies of the Commission's new COPPA privacy policy compliance guide, and were encouraged to call or e-mail the staff with any questions.

Rules on Obtaining Parental Consent

On October 31, 2001, the FTC published its proposal to extend the Rule's sliding scale mechanism for obtaining parental consent, originally slated to expire on April 21, 2002. Under the sliding scale, a Web site collecting personal information solely for its internal use, and not disclosing the information to the public or third parties, may obtain parental consent through the use of an e-mail message from the parent, coupled with additional steps to provide assurance that it is the parent providing the consent. If the Web site is going to disclose the personal information to the public or third parties, the Rule requires that the Web site use more reliable methods.

As part of the rulemaking process, the FTC sought comment on several questions, including the current and anticipated availability and affordability of secure electronic mechanisms and/or infomediary services for obtaining parental consent. The Commission also sought comment on the length of the proposed extension and the negative impact, if any, of extending the sliding scale mechanism.

The comments received indicated that secure electronic technology and infomediary services are not yet widely available at a reasonable cost and that the sliding scale mechanism to date has been an effective method for obtaining parental consent.

Accordingly, the FTC has extended the sliding scale mechanism for three years, until April 21, 2005. The Commission will re-examine this issue through public notice and comment in connection with the statutorily mandated review of the Rule in 2005.

14

Children Should Have Fewer First Amendment Rights than Adults

Kevin W. Saunders

Law professor Kevin W. Saunders is the author of Saving Our Children from the First Amendment, *which advocates for restricting advertising and violent, profane, or offensive expression.*

The capacities of children are different from those of adults, and the government should acknowledge this by granting fewer First Amendment liberties to minors. Because youths are unable to sufficiently judge what is or is not in their own best interests, the government must limit children's access to material that may negatively influence them, such as advertising, violent video games, and hate-filled music. These restrictions would help to alleviate the deleterious effects of media, which encourage minors to drink, smoke, have sex, and commit violent acts. Although often opposed by Americans, the suppression of speech is clearly necessary in order to protect children from harm until they turn eighteen, when their individual rights can and should be fully realized.

In 1949, Justice [Robert H.] Jackson wrote: "There is danger that, if the Court does not temper its doctrinaire logic with a little practical wisdom, it will convert the constitutional Bill of Rights into a suicide pact." Similarly, writing for the Court in 1963, Justice [Arthur] Goldberg stated: "[W]hile the Constitution protects against invasions of individual rights, it is not a suicide pact." The position that the Constitution is not a suicide pact finds support in other opinions of the Supreme Court and lower courts.

> *Rather than conclude that the rights of children and adults should be equal, [we should consider] limiting children's rights to correspond to children's capacities.*

Yet, how better for a society to commit suicide than to fail in its duty to raise its youth in a safe and psychologically healthy manner? We are so failing. While rates fluctuate, violent crime by youths is unacceptably high. Homicide is the second leading cause of death for 15- to 24-year-olds and the leading cause among African-American males of that age. Teenage pregnancy rates are also too high. Although down 11 percent from its 1994 high, the birth rate for unwed 15- to 19-year-olds was 41.5 births per thousand in 1998. Children also use tobacco and alcohol at unacceptable rates. The Campaign for Tobacco Free Kids cites government reports showing that more than 4 million 12- to 17-year-olds are current smokers, and 48.2 percent of high school boys used tobacco in the month preceding a 1997 survey. The Campaign for Alcohol Free Kids reports that 10 million American teenagers drink monthly; that 8 million drink weekly, a half million of those binge drinking; that alcohol consumption is not uncommon at ages 11 and 12; and that a majority of grade five through twelve students say that advertising encourages them to drink. We are failing in our duty to society and its coming generations, and the First Amendment's limitations on our ability to restrict the influences children face are among the roots of that failure.

The Rights of Children and Adults Are Not Equal

The First Amendment does contain the most important of our political freedoms. Stating those freedoms very succinctly, the amendment says: "Congress shall make no law respecting an establishment of religion, or prohibiting the free exercise thereof; or abridging the freedom of speech, or of the press; or the right of the people peaceably to assemble, and to petition the Government for a redress of grievances." The importance of the amendment for adults is obvious, but its importance for children is less clear. Even if children should enjoy some First Amendment rights, the benefits those rights provide may well be limited by a child's developmental stage. Rather than conclude that the rights of children and adults should be equal, the possibility of limiting children's rights to correspond to children's capacities should be considered.

Free expression also has its costs. While there are limitations on adult expression, those limitations are narrow. Only when a clear and present danger attends the speech or when the speech falls within certain categories—obscenity, fighting words, or libel—may adult speech be limited. When the recipient of the speech is a child still developing psychologically, the costs of unrestrained speech may be too high. Shielding children from harm adults may have to tolerate protects children in their development. This same shielding also serves to protect the rest of society. Any negative effects free expression has on children affect not only children but society as a whole.

> *// Courts make it very difficult to limit the access of children to . . . vulgar or profane materials, and the hate-filled music used to recruit the next generation to supremacist organizations. //*

The thesis of this article is that the First Amendment should function differently for children and for adults. For communication among adults, the amendment should be fully robust, perhaps even more so than under current law. Where children are concerned, however, the amendment should be significantly weaker. Society should be allowed to limit the access of children to materials not suitable to their age. Most people might be surprised to learn that the two-tiered approach to the First Amendment that I am proposing would generally be considered a departure from existing interpretations; at the moment, courts make it very difficult to limit the access of children to violent materials, vulgar or profane materials, and the hate-filled music used to recruit the next generation to supremacist organizations. Legal prohibitions on distributing sexual materials to children are now constitutional, and my approach would extend this treatment to the materials listed above. No good reason requires that we recognize a right on the part of children to such access. Nor should the free expression rights of adults be seen as including a right to express themselves to the children of others. The full development and autonomy of adults may require the right to express themselves on a wide variety of topics, but that right should not include access to children not their own. Perhaps no one should tell authors, producers, or computer programmers what they can create. But that is not the same as saying that they have a right to a juvenile audience for their books, films, or video games.

The Enforcement of Morality Is Often Opposed

Those who argue for strong individual rights or autonomy consider the imposition of morality through the law illegitimate, but it is important to understand the nature of the objections. However complex or sophisticated the way in which the argument is presented, it seems to come down to the complaint that society's attempt to enforce morality is paternalistic. That is, when the state forbids behavior that only affects consenting, competent participants, the only basis for the intervention is the state's belief that it knows better than the individual what is best for that individual. There are, of course, contingent arguments over who is affected by the behavior, but the jurisprudential issue is over the right of the state to limit the individual's ability to make decisions having an effect solely on that individual.

> *While obscenity laws continue to exist, their enforcement has become more lax and the likelihood that a particular work will be found obscene has decreased.*

When the charge of paternalism is raised against a proscription regarding adult behavior, it has some impact. Clearly, it would further the individual's own best health interests if the state were to forbid smoking. But our society believes that individuals should be able to make their own decisions in such cases. The same applies to the use of alcohol, although drug laws seem to indicate the limits of the culture's receptiveness to such autonomy arguments.

[Paternalism] may be inappropriate when the action is toward an adult, but it is completely appropriate when a father or mother acts that way toward his or her child.

When it comes to issues of free expression, the antipaternalistic feeling is particularly strong. Through the first half of the 20th century, adult use of obscene materials was routinely suppressed, largely on the theory that such use was not good for the individual. While obscenity laws continue to exist, their enforcement has become more lax and the likelihood that a particular work will be found obscene has decreased. The decreasing acceptability of paternalism was central in *Stanley v. Georgia*. In that case, the Supreme Court reversed a conviction for the possession of obscene materials in the privacy of the defendant's home. The state argued that it had the right to protect the mind of the individual from the effect of obscenity, but the Court flatly rejected the claim, concluding that "if the First Amendment means anything, it means that a State has no business telling a man, sitting alone in his own house, what books he may read or what films he may watch." The Court went on to say that the state "cannot constitutionally premise legislation on the desirability of controlling a person's private thoughts."

Youths Need Protection and Guidance

Since many arguments against restrictions on free expression, like many arguments against the enforcement of morality generally, are based on antipaternalistic feelings, it is important to understand just what is wrong with paternalism. Paternalism, when it is wrong, is wrong because it is an affront to equality. When the state tells the individual what is in the individual's best interest, the state discounts the individual's own view as to how to balance his or her own interests. It treats the individual as less able to make such a decision than the majority the state represents, and numbers alone should not resolve such disagreements over individual goods.

Children, however, are not equals in this regard. Knowing what one's best interests are requires an ability to make judgments that children, depending on their age, may completely lack or that may be insufficiently developed in them. "Paternalism" means acting like a father. That may be inappropriate when the action is toward an adult, but it is completely appropriate when a father or mother acts that way toward his or her child. Children need to be taught how to act, both when the acts involved may have an effect on others and when the issue is what is in the child's own best interests. The same is true when the issue is what to read or see. There may be no right to interfere with an adult's decisions as to the materials he or she believes contribute to understanding or happiness. With children, however, it is appropriate for parents to decide what materials run counter to their child becoming the sort of person they think the child should be and to refuse to allow the child access to those materials.

> *Once a child reaches adulthood, individual rights can come into full bloom.*

The state also serves a role with regard to children that is, in a sense, parental. The state may act in its *parens patriae* role in a parental manner. When it does so, its role is paternalistic, but not in the pejorative sense in which the word is usually used. The role of the state, so long as the parents are not unfit, is secondary to the parents, but just as preventing non-parents from selling tobacco to minors is not objectionably paternalistic, limiting the ability of non-parents to distribute harmful media to children should not be objectionably paternalistic.

Protecting Children's Best Interests

Allowing the state to limit third party expression to children would enable society to promote good values without imposing majority views on or limiting the personal autonomy of adults. The community would have the period of the child's minority to transmit its values from generation to generation.

This fits with John Stuart Mill's own recognition that society has the period of childhood to teach its children how to act. At the same time, once a child reaches adulthood, individual rights can come into full bloom. Such individual rights may still interfere with or run counter to community values, but the community had its opportunity to teach those values. If it has failed to do so, the values may simply be of insufficient strength to override the commitment to individual rights society also recognizes.

> *" Children are, in fact, not equals, . . . [and] they need help in their development. "*

Society may have a right to make people morally better, but it has the period of minority to do so. Children must be trained, morally as well as in other areas. They need to be made into the morally best people they can be, but the project should be relatively complete by the time the child reaches the age of majority. To carry it on beyond that age is disrespectful of the equality of the individual. To engage in the task before the age of majority is to recognize that children are, in fact, not equals, in a sense, and that they need help in their development. The acceptance of a strong First Amendment for adults and a weaker First Amendment for children would allow society to protect children's best interests as well as its own.

Violent Media Has Grave Effects on Children

The distribution of violent material such as videos and video games illustrates why the dual approach to the First Amendment makes sense. *Doom* is the best known of the "first-person shooter" genre of video games. In these games the player holds a realistic hand gun and fires at people who pop up or come around corners on the video screen. Killing quickly and efficiently produces high scores. The games are such good training that adaptations are used by the armed forces and law enforcement agencies. Most users, however, are not soldiers but teenage boys.

In 1997, Michael Carneal was a 14-year-old freshman at Heath High School in Paducah, Kentucky. He enjoyed playing

Doom and similar video games. He had also seen the film *The Basketball Diaries*, in which the film's hero, in a dream sequence, goes to school with a firearm under his trench coat and guns down a teacher and several classmates. One morning Carneal went to his school with a stolen pistol, arriving just as a prayer group was breaking up. He opened fire on the group and with nine shots inflicted head or chest wounds on eight students, killing three. He did so with no firearm experience other than on video games.

Two years later, Eric Harris and Dylan Klebold went to Columbine High School in Littleton, Colorado. They were heavily armed, and by the time they were finished and committed suicide, they had killed a teacher and 12 students and had wounded 23 others. They too were avid *Doom* players. . . .

Recognizing the difference between the free expression interests of adults and children only makes sense. The dual approach would be in the best interests of children and society.

Organizations to Contact

ABA Juvenile Justice Center
740 Fifteenth St. NW, 7th Fl., Washington, DC 20005
(202) 662-1506 • fax: (202) 662-1507
e-mail: juvjus@abanet.org • Web site: www.abanet.org

An organization of the American Bar Association, the Juvenile Justice Center disseminates information on juvenile justice systems and laws that pertain to youths. The center provides leadership to state and local practitioners, judges, youth workers, and policy makers on topics ranging from school zero tolerance policies to capital punishment of juveniles. Its publications include the quarterly *Criminal Justice Magazine*.

Advocates for Youth
2000 M St. NW, Suite 750, Washington, DC 20036
(202) 419-3420 • fax: (202) 419-1448
e-mail: questions@advocatesforyouth.org
Web site: www.advocatesforyouth.org

Advocates for Youth believes young people have the right to access information and services that help prevent teen pregnancy and the spread of sexually transmitted diseases. To enable youths to make healthy decisions about sexuality, the organization prints brochures, fact sheets, and bibliographies on adolescent pregnancy and sexuality, adolescent rights, and sexuality education. *Advocating for Adolescent Reproductive Health in Eastern Europe and Central Asia* is among its reports.

American Civil Liberties Union (ACLU)
125 Broad St., 18th Fl., New York, NY 10004-2400
(212) 549-2500
e-mail: aclu@aclu.org • Web site: www.aclu.org

The ACLU is a national organization that works to defend Americans' civil rights guaranteed by the U.S. Constitution. Its Freedom Wire division, which can be accessed on its Web site, provides information on the free speech, privacy, and reproductive rights of minors and students. The ACLU offers policy statements, pamphlets, a *Student Organizing Manual*, and the semiannual newsletter *Civil Liberties Alert*.

Amnesty International (AI)
5 Penn Plaza, 14th Fl., New York, NY 10001
(212) 807-8400 • fax: (212) 627-1451
e-mail: aimember@aiusa.org • Web site: www.amnesty.org

Amnesty International is a worldwide independent movement that works to free people detained for their beliefs, ethnic origin, sex, language, economic status, birth, or other status. The children's rights link on its Web site offers access to a number of briefings and reports on child soldiery, circumcision, and the execution of juveniles. AI also publishes a quarterly newsletter titled *Amnesty International*.

Bureau of International Labor Affairs (ILAB)
U.S. Department of Labor
200 Constitution Ave. NW, Room S-2235, Washington, DC 20210
(202) 219-6061
Web site: www.dol.gov/dol/ilab

ILAB carries out the U.S. Department of Labor's international responsibilities and assists in formulating the international economic, trade, and immigration policies that affect American workers. Its reports on child labor include *By the Sweat and Toil of Children* and *The Apparel Industry and Codes of Conduct: A Solution to the International Child Labor Problem?*

Cato Institute
1000 Massachusetts Ave. NW, Washington, DC 20001-5403
(202) 842-0200 • fax: (202) 842-3490
Web site: www.cato.org

The Cato Institute is a libertarian public policy research foundation dedicated to limiting the role of government and protecting individual liberties. Some of the many topics it discusses include labor, Internet privacy, and inefficiency and abuse in America's schools. The institute produces the quarterly magazine *Regulation*, the bimonthly *Cato Policy Report*, numerous books, and various policy papers and articles, including *Child Labor or Child Prostitution?*

Children's Rights
404 Park Ave. South, 11th Fl., New York, New York 10016
(212) 683-2210
e-mail: info@childrensrights.org • Web site: www.childrensrights.org

Children's Rights promotes the rights of abused and neglected children in U.S. foster care. Using policy analysis, public education and the power of the courts, the organization works to reform the child welfare system and ensure that children are kept safe and healthy. On its Web site Children's Rights makes available press releases, legal briefings, and other publications, such as *Winning for Children: Using the Courts to Reform Child Welfare.*

Child Welfare League of America (CWLA)
440 First St. NW, Suite 310, Washington, DC 20001-2085
(202) 638-2952 • fax: (202) 638-4004
Web site: www.cwla.org

The Child Welfare League is an association of more than seven hundred public and private agencies and organizations devoted to improving the lives of children. CWLA publishes the journal *Child Welfare* six times a year, *Children's Voice* quarterly, and more than twenty books a year. Its areas of interest include adolescent pregnancy, child abuse and neglect, foster care, and the juvenile justice system.

Family Research Council (FRC)
801 G St. NW, Washington, DC 20001
(202) 393-2100 • fax: (202) 393-2134
Web site: www.frc.org

The council seeks to promote and protect the interests of the traditional family, concentrating on issues such as parental autonomy and responsibility, community support for single parents, and adolescent pregnancy. FRC opposes the Convention on the Rights of the Child and supports capital punishment of juveniles. "Abstinence Until Marriage: The Best Message for Teens" is one of the council's papers.

Global Exchange
2017 Mission St., No. 303, San Francisco, CA 94110
(415) 255-7296 • (800) 497-1994 • fax: (415) 255-7498
e-mail: gx-info@globalexchange.org
Web site: www.globalexchange.org

Global Exchange is a nonprofit organization that promotes social justice, environmental sustainability, and grassroots activism on international human rights issues. The group produces various books, videos, and other educational programs and materials concerning human rights. Its Web site contains a link for sweatshops.

Heritage Foundation
214 Massachusetts Ave. NE, Washington, DC 20002
(202) 546-4400 • fax: (202) 546-8328
e-mail: info@heritage.org • Web site: www.heritage.org

The Heritage Foundation is a conservative public policy research institute that advocates free-market economics and limited government. Education, welfare reform, and labor laws are three of the many issues it addresses. Publications of the Heritage Foundation include the monthly *Policy Review*, the Backgrounder series of papers, and the Heritage Lectures series.

Human Rights Watch (HRW)
485 Fifth Ave., New York, NY 10017-6104
(212) 972-8400 • fax: (212) 972-0905
e-mail: hrwnyc@hrw.org • Web site: www.hrw.org

Human Rights Watch investigates human rights abuses in over seventy countries around the world. It promotes civil liberties and defends freedom of thought, due process, and the equal protection of the law. A children's rights link on its Web site directs readers to news releases, other links, and countless reports, including *Future Forsaken: Abuses Against Children Affected by HIV/AIDS in India*. HRW also prints the *Human Rights Watch Quarterly Newsletter* and the annual *Human Rights Watch World Report*.

International Labour Office (ILO)
Washington Branch, 1828 L St. NW, Washington, DC 20036
(202) 653-7652 • fax: (202) 653-7687
e-mail: washington@ilo.org • e-mail: ilo@ilo.org
Web site: www.ilo.org

The ILO works to promote basic human rights through improved working and living conditions and by enhancing opportunities for those who are excluded from meaningful salaried employment. It runs the ILO Publications Bureau, which publishes various policy statements and background information on all aspects of employment. *Child Labour: Targeting the Intolerable* is an ILO publication.

United Nations Children's Fund (UNICEF)
National Committee, 333 E. Thirty-eighth St., New York, NY 10016
(212) 686-5522 • fax: (212) 779-1679
e-mail: information@unicefusa.org
Web site: www.unicef.org • Web site: www.unicefusa.org

The United States is one of 37 nations that raises money for UNICEF, an organization that provides health care, clean water, improved nutrition, and education to millions of children in more than 160 countries and territories. UNICEF also works to spread awareness about the status of the world's children. Among its publications are *The State of the World's Children 2005, Early Marriage: A Harmful Traditional Practice*, and presentation papers from international child welfare and labor conferences.

Bibliography

Books

David Archard — *Children: Rights and Childhood.* London: Routledge, 2004.

Kathleen Conn — *The Internet and the Law: What Educators Need to Know.* Alexandria, VA: Association for Supervision and Curriculum Development, 2002.

Kerry Kennedy Cuomo — *Truth to Power: Human Rights Defenders Who Are Changing Our World.* New York: Crown, 2000.

Mark Ensalaco — *Children's Human Rights: Progress and Challenges for Children Worldwide.* Lanham, MD, and Boulder, CO: Rowman & Littlefield, 2005.

Martin Guggenheim — *What's Wrong with Children's Rights?* Cambridge, MA: Harvard University Press, 2005.

Kay S. Hymowitz — *Ready or Not: Why Treating Children as Small Adults Endangers Their Future—and Ours.* New York: Free Press, 1999.

International Programme on the Elimination of Child Labour (IPEC) — *Child Labour Book 1: Children's Rights and Education.* Geneva, Switzerland: International Labour Office, 2003.

Peter Irons, ed. — *May It Please the Court: Courts, Kids, and the Constitution.* New York: New Press, 2000.

Baba Jallow — *Dying for My Daughter.* San Anselmo, CA, and Hillview, KY: Wasteland Press, 2004.

Kay Ann Johnson — *Wanting a Daughter, Needing a Son: Abandonment, Adoption, and Orphanage Care in China.* Edited by Amy Klatzkin. St. Paul, MN: Yeong & Yeong, 2004.

Jonathan Kozol — *Ordinary Resurrections: Children in the Years of Hope.* New York: Crown, 2000.

Nicholas D. Kristof and Sheryl WuDunn — *Thunder from the East: Portrait of a Rising Asia.* New York: Knopf, 2000.

Marvin J. Levine — *Children for Hire: The Perils of Child Labor in the United States.* Westport, CT: Praeger, 2003.

Duncan Lindsey — *The Welfare of Children.* Oxford, UK: Oxford University Press, 2003.

Susan Linn — *Consuming Kids: The Hostile Takeover of Childhood.* New York: New Press, 2004.

Charles S. McCoy, ed.   *Promises to Keep: Prospects for Human Rights*. Berkeley, CA: Center for Ethics and Social Policy, Graduate Theological Union, and Literary Directions, 2002.

John T. Pardeck   *Children's Rights: Policy and Practice*. New York: Haworth Social Work, 2002.

Robert C. Prall   *The Rights of Children in Separation and Divorce*. Kansas City, MO: Landmark Editions, 2000.

Jamin B. Raskin   *We the Students: Supreme Court Decisions for and About Students*. Washington, DC: CQ Press, 2003.

Diane Ravitch and Joseph P. Viteritti, eds.   *Kid Stuff: Marketing Sex and Violence to America's Children*. Baltimore: Johns Hopkins University Press, 2003.

Jeremy Seabrook   *Children of Other Worlds: Exploitation in the Global Market*. London: Pluto Press, 2001.

Traci Truly   *Teen Rights: A Legal Guide for Teens and the Adults in Their Lives*. Naperville, IL: Sphinx, 2002.

Virginia A. Walter   *Children and Libraries: Getting It Right*. Chicago: American Library Association, 2000.

Periodicals

Sasha Abramsky   "Taking Juveniles Off Death Row," *American Prospect*, July 2004.

Joe Blankenau and Mark Leeper   "Public School Search Policies and the 'Politics of Sin,'" *Policy Studies Journal*, November 2003.

Bruce Bower   "Teen Brains on Trial: The Science of Neural Development Tangles with the Juvenile Death Penalty," *Science News*, May 8, 2004.

Margaret Brazier   "Right-to-Die Disputes," *Hospital Doctor*, November 18, 2004.

Vasana Chinvarakorn   "Where Have All the Children Gone? Gone to the Graveyards or Sweatshops, as the Numbers of Child Soldiers and Labourers Increase," *Bangkok Post*, February 19, 2001.

Abigail English and Carol A. Ford   "The HIPAA Privacy Rule and Adolescents: Legal Questions and Clinical Challenges," *Perspectives on Sexual and Reproductive Health*, March/April 2004.

Bruce C. Hafen and Jonathan O. Hafen   "Abandoning Children to Their Rights," *First Things*, August/September 1995.

Mary Renck Jalongo   "The Child's Right to Creative Thought and Expression," *Childhood Education*, Summer 2003.

Rachel Johnson   "Bum Rap Pinned On Parents," *Spectator*, May 29, 2004.

Peter Kreeft	"The Apple Argument Against Abortion," *Crisis*, December 2000.
Nicholas D. Kristof	"Inviting All Democrats," *New York Times*, January 14, 2004.
Stephen McGarvey	"Safeguarding Sovereignty," *Home School Court Report*, November/December 2002.
Moira Rayner	"Resilience, Refugees, and the Rights of Children—an Immorality Play," *Psychiatry, Psychology and Law*, November 2004.
Stephen N. Roberts	"Tracking Your Children with GPS: Do You Have the Right?" *Wireless Business & Technology*, December 2003.
Richard Rothstein	"Defending Sweatshops: Too Much Logic, Too Little Evidence," *Dissent*, Spring 2005.
Peter Singer	"Pulling Back the Curtain on the Mercy Killing of Newborns," *Los Angeles Times*, March 11, 2005.
Don Sloan	"The Shame of Child Labor," *Political Affairs*, January 2005.
Ashley A. Smith	"Young Voices: Teenagers Have Adult Reasons to Vote," *Detroit Free Press*, August 23, 2004.
Toronto Star	"Don't Rush Voting Right," March 25, 2005.
Keith Wade	"The Internet: Parental Guidance Preferred," *Freeman*, February 2000.

Internet Sources

Administration for Children and Families	*A Childhood for Every Child: How Compassion-Driven Solutions are Transforming the Nation's Well-Being.* Department of Health and Human Services, 2005. www.acf.hhs.gov.
Amnesty International	"Cote D'Ivoire—Stop the Use of Child Soldiers," March 18, 2005. www.amnesty.org.
Anti-Slavery Society	"Child Labor in the Carpet Industry," 2003. www.antislaverysociety.addr.com.
Chris B.	"Capital Punishment for Youth," Ink Droppings. www.m-a-h.net.
Jennifer S. Butler	"Myths and Realities About the UN's Work with Women and Children," Ecumenical Women 2000+. www.ew2000plus.org.
Andy Carvin	"Student Free Speech Rights on the Internet and the Ghosts of Columbine," *Digital Beat*, April 20, 2000. www.benton.org.
Electoral Commission	*Age of Electoral Majority*. April 19, 2004. www.electoralcommission.org.uk.

Tanya L. Green	"Not in My School," *Family Voice*, March/April 2001. www.cwfa.org.
Human Rights Watch	*Borderline Slavery: Child Trafficking in Togo.* 2003. www.hrw.org.
Human Rights Watch	*"You'll Learn Not to Cry": Child Combatants in Colombia.* September 2003. www.hrw.org.
Muslim Women's League	"Female Genital Mutilation," January 1999. www.mwlusa.org.
Jordan Riak	*Plain Talk About Spanking.* Parents and Teachers Against Violence in Education, August 2002. www.nospank.net
Melissa Sickmund	*Juveniles in Corrections.* Office of Juvenile Justice and Delinquency Prevention, June 2004. www.ncjrs.org.
United Nations	Convention on the Rights of the Child, November 20, 1989. www.unhchr.ch.
United Nations Children's Fund (UNICEF)	*All Rights for All Children.* January 2005. www.unicef.org.

Index